W9-CNN-644

DATE DUE

PREVENTING DRUG ABUSE

What do we know?

Dean R. Gerstein and Lawrence W. Green, *editors*

Committee on Drug Abuse Prevention Research

Commission on Behavioral and Social Sciences and Education

National Research Council

NATIONAL ACADEMY PRESS
Washington, D.C.   1993

National Academy Press • 2101 Constitution Avenue, N.W. • Washington, D.C. 20418

NOTICE: The project that is the subject of this report was approved by the Governing Board of the National Research Council, whose members are drawn from the councils of the National Academy of Sciences, the National Academy of Engineering, and the Institute of Medicine. The members of the committee responsible for the report were chosen for their special competences and with regard for appropriate balance.

This report has been reviewed by a group other than the authors according to procedures approved by a Report Review Committee consisting of members of the National Academy of Sciences, the National Academy of Engineering, and the Institute of Medicine.

This project was sponsored by the National Institute on Drug Abuse.

Library of Congress Cataloging-in-Publication Data

Preventing drug abuse : what do we know? / Dean R. Gerstein and
    Lawrence W. Green, editors.
    p.   cm
   Includes bibliographical references and index.
   ISBN 0-309-04627-0
   1. Drug abuse—United States. 2. Drug abuse —United States—
Prevention—Evaluation. I. Gerstein, Dean R. II. Green, Lawrence W.
HV5825.P74   1993   93-7333
362.29'17'0973—dc20   CIP

COMMITTEE ON DRUG ABUSE PREVENTION RESEARCH

*Resigned in 1990.

The National Academy of Sciences is a private, nonprofit, self-perpetuating society of distinguished scholars engaged in scientific and engineering research, dedicated to the furtherance of science and technology and to their use for the general welfare. Upon the authority of the charter granted to it by the Congress in 1863, the Academy has a mandate that requires it to advise the federal government on scientific and technical matters. Dr. Frank Press is president of the National Academy of Sciences.

The National Academy of Engineering was established in 1964, under the charter of the National Academy of Sciences, as a parallel organization of outstanding engineers. It is autonomous in its administration and in the selection of its members, sharing with the National Academy of Sciences the responsibility for advising the federal government. The National Academy of Engineering also sponsors engineering programs aimed at meeting national needs, encourages education and research, and recognizes the superior achievements of engineers. Dr. Robert M. White is president of the National Academy of Engineering.

The Institute of Medicine was established in 1970 by the National Academy of Sciences to secure the services of eminent members of appropriate professions in the examination of policy matters pertaining to the health of the public. The Institute acts under the responsibility given to the National Academy of Sciences by its congressional charter to be an adviser to the federal government and, upon its own initiative, to identify issues of medical care, research, and education. Dr. Kenneth I. Shine is president of the Institute of Medicine.

The National Research Council was organized by the National Academy of Sciences in 1916 to associate the broad community of science and technology with the Academy's purposes of furthering knowledge and advising the federal government. Functioning in accordance with general policies determined by the Academy, the Council has become the principal operating agency of both the National Academy of Sciences and the National Academy of Engineering in providing services to the government, the public, and the scientific and engineering communities. The Council is administered jointly by both Academies and the Institute of Medicine. Dr. Frank Press and Dr. Robert M. White are chairman and vice chairman, respectively, of the National Research Council.

Contents

Preface

The task of developing scientific knowledge relevant to drug abuse prevention has been a distinct item on the public health research agenda for several decades. The National Institute on Drug Abuse (NIDA), which evolved from a division within the National Institute of Mental Health, has sponsored extramural research on prevention-related topics at the rate of several million dollars annually since the mid-1970s. In the 1980s, other research agencies of the federal government, such as the Centers for Disease Control, the Department of Education, and the Department of Justice, have intensified their interest in this topic. NIDA's sister agency in the Public Health Service, the Center for Substance Abuse Prevention, has obligated very substantial sums to a large number of demonstration projects, from which it is hoped that useful evaluation data may be expected. Moreover, a number of private foundations and state and local government agencies have committed very significant resources to new drug abuse prevention activities that entail research or program evaluation components.

Tangible progress in prevention research combined with substantially increased interest in prevention program evaluations and demonstration led NIDA to ask the National Research Council for assistance in shaping its own research agenda and providing certain common scientific reference points for others who are interested in the prevention research enterprise. That request led to the formation of the Committee on Drug Abuse Prevention Research and to this report of the committee.

The charge to the committee was not an open-ended or comprehensive review of the broad front of prevention policies and strategies. Rather, the committee followed a research-oriented agenda covering the following specific points of interest to NIDA:

Review the current status of drug abuse prevention research:

•   Assess the theoretical basis for preventive interventions as derived from etiologic research.

•   Identify which drug abuse prevention strategies have been adequately evaluated and found to be effective, not effective, and counter-effective (i.e., those that actually encourage drug abuse).

•   For drug abuse prevention strategies that have been found to be effective, assess how practical are such strategies for use in wide-scale applications and with other population groups (e.g., minorities).

•   Identify which prevention strategies have unknown effectiveness because of inadequate evaluation (e.g., insufficient numbers of replications).

Review methodological issues regarding drug abuse prevention strategies:

•   Identify major design and methodology problems in existing prevention strategies (i.e., inappropriate control groups, high or nonrandom subject attrition rates, problems with verification or self-report of drug use, contamination by other preventive interventions).

•   Identify possible approaches for correcting such problems in current and future prevention research.

•   Identify minimum requirements for assessing effectiveness of prevention strategies.

NIDA also invited the committee to offer recommendations, as appropriate, concerning the directions of future research.

The charge to the committee specified that it should focus on illicit drug problems. This limitation was not intended to downplay the public health importance of alcohol and tobacco but to assure that maximum guidance would be obtained for the central research mission of NIDA. The committee therefore considered research on prevention of alcohol and tobacco abuse only to the extent that this research is relevant to preventing illicit drug problems. The fact that alcohol and tobacco are generally illicit *for minors* creates an irreducible overlap in prevention concepts and interventions for young people.

We note that a committee at the Institute of Medicine of the National Academy of Sciences has completed a separate study of research needs and opportunities on alcohol problems (*Prevention and Treatment of Alcohol Problems: Research Opportunities*, Institute of Medicine, 1989), which provided much more comprehensive attention to alcohol abuse prevention as such.

In responding to NIDA's request, the National Research Council appointed a committee of research experts from a range of relevant disciplines, who reviewed the portfolio of current research and considered the lessons to be drawn for each item in the charge. This report, the result of the committee's deliberations, is organized into three chapters, which cover: the nature of the drug problems, particularly in terms of etiologic and epidemiologic data; the conceptual and theoretical foundations of research-based prevention interventions; and the evaluation of prevention programs' effectiveness.

The role of community channels and settings for drug abuse prevention seemed to us valuable in illuminating an important direction of research in which an expanded, methodologically sophisticated increment of attention is needed. With the partial exception of research on cigarette smoking, there has not been much attention in drug abuse research to the literature on community health education. We therefore include here an appendix on community strategies of health promotion and disease prevention, emphasizing the importance of implementation planning in making prevention programs sustainable.

We are particularly indebted to two committee members, Patrick O'Malley and Richard Clayton, who took on more than a usual share of the work in drafting the chapters of this report. We would also like to acknowledge the help of Ralph Tarter, who participated in two committee meetings and Carol Weiss, who participated in one; Herbert Kleber and Mary Ann Pentz, who gave stimulating presentations at respective meetings; Zili Amsel and William Bukoski, the NIDA project officers; and the dedicated panel of anonymous reviewers appointed by the National Research Council.

The committee owes much to the Commission on Behavioral and Social Sciences and Eduation, particularly Eugenia Grohman, associate director of reports, who provided administrative guidance and support; Christine McShane, editor without peer, who groomed the text and brought it through the final stages of preparation; Linda Kearney, administrative coordinator of the study; and Elaine McGarraugh, who served throughout as assistant study director—compiling and organizing research materials, drafting parts of the report, and generally ensuring its progress and completion. Margaret Cargo, research assistant at the University of British Columbia, assisted in the final rounds of bibliographic and data compilation.

Lawrence W. Green, *Chair*
Dean R. Gerstein, *Study Director*

PREVENTING DRUG ABUSE

What do we know?

Executive Summary

In an expansive view of the drug problem, drug abuse prevention research could be seen as a burgeoning domain, encompassing nearly every type of research with a bearing on individual health and social well-being, from the molecular to the global. However, the purview of this report is not nearly so expansive. Its purpose is threefold:

- Assess the self-designated drug abuse prevention strategies that have been subjects of evaluation research, which are limited largely to a few domains of health-oriented interventions;
- Consider the explicit theoretical basis and methodological adequacy of these evaluation findings and assess their applicability to diverse population segments; and
- Proffer minimum methodological standards for future evaluation projects.

Within this scope, as defined by the sponsor of the study, the National Institute on Drug Abuse (NIDA), the committee has framed a limited set of conclusions concerning the direction of future research. The literature reviewed in this report is devoted nearly entirely to studies of youth under age 20 and psychoactive drugs that are illegal for young people to purchase: the fully illicit drugs such as marijuana, heroin, and crack cocaine; the "prescription-only" drugs such as barbiturates and amphetamines; and the "adults-only" drugs, cigarettes and alcohol.

The following summary responses to the specific points of NIDA's charge reflect our reading of this literature in the light shed by scientific principles, keeping in mind the pragmatic challenges of conducting research with human subjects in real social institutions on a topic bristling with emotional and political thorns.

Review the current status of drug abuse prevention research; assess the theoretical basis for preventive interventions as derived from etiologic research.

Research on drug abuse prevention is haunted by a double vision that emerges from epidemiologic studies. There seem to be two worlds of drug abuse. In one world, that of relatively low-intensity consumption (drug *use*) among individuals who can be found in schools and households, drug experience is self-reported more frequently by the wealthy than the less wealthy and by whites than Hispanics or blacks. In this world, there have been steady and cumulatively very marked declines in the prevalence of marijuana use since the late 1970s and of cocaine since the middle 1980s, and heroin use is so rare as to be barely measurable. In another world, that of emergency rooms, morgues, drug clinics, juvenile detention centers, jails, and prisons, in which indicators of intensive drug consumption (*abuse* and *dependence*) are collected: the poor predominate, blacks and Hispanics appearing in numbers much higher than their household or school proportions; marijuana and heroin use are common (though less so in some areas than in the 1970s); and cocaine use increased explosively throughout the 1980s and simply leveled off at high levels in the 1990s.

The validity of the data that define each of these worlds, although subject to some degree of error and drift, is beyond knowledgeable dispute. Reconciling the two worlds in terms of theoretical understanding and empirical mechanisms, however, is a major research issue. To some degree these discrepancies may represent time lags, as tidal changes in the social acceptability and marketing of illicit drugs work their way through age-specific multiyear developmental pathways that lead from more or less common experimental use to a much smaller residual core of chronic drug dependence. But more of the discrepancy appears attributable to deep-seated divisions between the circumstances and social reinforcements of rich and poor, ethnic/linguistic majorities and minorities, and individuals predisposed toward or against strong attachments to drug-taking behaviors even before the opportunities to use specific drugs arise.

A major finding of etiologic research is that the onset of drug taking follows relatively orderly sequences, which begin in early adolescence with the illicit use of alcohol and tobacco—drugs widely and legally available to adults although prohibited to minors—and end for some in a glut of drug consumption including the above and extending to cocaine and possibly heroin. For this reason, efforts to stop or at least delay to older ages the onset of use of these drugs, as well as efforts to act directly against marijuana and cocaine use, are suggestive paths for interventions. However, etiologic research also gives strong reasons to think that early onset can mean very different things for youths whose social supports are strong and relatively untroubled, than for those whose social environment is impoverished or antagonistic and whose behavior includes a substantial repertoire of illegal and hazardous activities.

As a result, the research suggests that prevention may need to proceed along distinct paths and that interventions may prove to have contradictory effects—null for some, appreciable for others, even negative as well as positive directions of change in desired outcomes for different subpopulations. Etiologic studies further tell us that these populations are sorted and shaped in their knowledge, attitudes, and behavior by the people in whose presence (both personal and impersonal) they spend their lives. There is, in particular, a substantial deficit of information about how schools and communities—two major youth-affecting institutions—do this shaping and sorting, and how preventive interventions delivered person-to-person and through mass communications media interlock with the dynamic life of schools and communities. Strategic research initiatives are needed to improve our understanding of the normative and economic aspects of communities and the normative and socioenvironmental character of schools and other institutions, as they affect drug-related and other health behavior, in order to prime the next generation of prevention strategies.

Identify which drug abuse prevention strategies have been adequately evaluated and found to be effective, not effective, and countereffective.

On balance, we conclude that no drug abuse prevention activities have been adequately evaluated and found to be reliably effective, in all cases, with all groups. One near-exception arises, in which a critical mass of findings of effectiveness are vitiated by methodological doubts and tempered by questions about the persistence and homogeneity of observed effects: interventions in school settings from the 6th through 10th grades, focusing on behavioral training of skills to assertively counteract or resist (and, implicitly, to desist from exerting) explicit peer pressure toward use, lodged within a more general curriculum emphasizing self-efficacy, interpersonal social skills, and specific knowledge of health effects, followed up with booster sessions in a subsequent school year, and concomitant with continuing public health efforts on a community-wide basis, have in a notable number of trials been effective *in delaying the onset of cigarette smoking* for a sizable fraction of students who would otherwise have begun smoking early in their adolescence.

Although this seems a consistent enough finding to merit notice, there are important codicils. In controlled experimental studies begun long enough ago to yield follow-ups of 5 years or more, the deceleration in onset of cigarette smoking by students in the first year or more after exposure to the intervention does not necessarily yield lower smoking rates by the time students reach the upper classes of high school. Later interventions, using more technically refined approaches, may or may not prove to sustain these effects. However, even a delay in onset of smoking is noteworthy. Cigarette smokers who begin smoking later are likely to quit smoking sooner, and if smoking precedes onset of other drugs, later smoking means later onset of other drugs for which similar patterns (start later—quit sooner) apply.

More troubling about these studies are indications that the effects are not uniform; in exemplary, rigorously controlled evaluation, the students who had *already begun smoking* before receiving the curriculum became *more likely* to continue smoking afterward, even though the students who had *not begun smoking* were *less likely* to start afterward. The rates of attrition in these studies, particularly due to their reliance on school-based sampling, leave these subgroup results somewhat unsettled. Nevertheless, these negative findings point to *counter*effectiveness within the subpopulation described earlier as the second world of etiologic risk, and the positive results match findings elsewhere supporting effectiveness with the first-world population.

Some prevention strategies have been evaluated sufficiently to conclude that they are *not* widely effective. The will to believe on the part of implementers and program sponsors alike seems stronger than the evidence supports. This applies in particular to those school-based activities that do not at any point deal directly with the training of behavior between peers, but rather focus only on increasing knowledge about health effects, improving interpersonal skills, or improving feelings of self-esteem.

For drug abuse prevention strategies that have been found to be effective, assess how practical such strategies are for use in wide-scale applications and with other population groups (i.e., minorities).

Because we cannot count any strategies as clearly and consistently effective, the committee considers this point moot. Wide-scale programs must be conceived and executed as multiple strategies, each tailored to the specific population group it seeks to influence.

Identify which prevention strategies have unknown effectiveness because of inadequate evaluation (i.e., insufficient numbers of replications).

Although no inventory of prevention strategies has been taken that would identify the largest absorbers of funding, several school-based, skills-training-inclusive curricula (in particular, DARE and the Here's Looking at You series) are so widely employed that we must recommend the completion of additional rigorous evaluations by independent researchers—or these strategies should cease being used.

Were resources unlimited, we could well call for generous ladles of funding to support more and better evaluations of a substantial range of other intervention approaches. However, we find that, on the whole, an insufficient number of replications is not the main obstacle to identifying effective strategies. There seems much more warrant for formative, relatively smaller-scale studies—using trials and other methodologies—of prevention strategies based on theoretical principles such as risk-factor reduction and developmental shaping of behavior. At the same time, broad-scale community strategies and conditions of living need research attention, for it is within the broader community context that any school-based or other strategy must operate and trace its effects.

> **Review methodological issues regarding drug abuse prevention strategies: identify major design and methodology problems in evaluating existing prevention strategies and possible approaches for correcting such problems in current and future prevention research.**

A clear majority of the research published as evaluations of the effectiveness of preventive interventions is methodologically weak. To a certain degree, this is an unsurprising result of imbalance between the large volume of prevention-oriented activities and the modest volume of support for their evaluation. A catalog of these weaknesses would be tiresome and perhaps misleading—there are a respectable number of sound studies. However, the most common, fundamental problems, which afflict even some of the most widely cited research, are as follows:

• Cursory description and documentation of the intervention methods, the evaluation designs, the outcome measures used, and the characteristics of treatment and control populations, in terms of both personal characteristics and social circumstances.
• Partial or missing measurement of instrumental processes and intermediate and final effects, including individual exposure to materials, messages, or training; retention of knowledge; acceptance of affective or attitudinal impressions; changes in assertive or other behavior; changes in levels of drug consumption; changes in drug-related sequelae.
• No attention to concurrent prevention activities in the experimental or control locales.
• Inadequate follow-up, insufficient time frames, and response rates that are too low and subject to serious biases.

The correction of such issues, insofar as that is within the power of NIDA, is not a matter of applying rigid formulae. It requires a patient commitment to attracting quality researchers to the field; applying requirements such as discussed below to NIDA publications and encouraging other research sponsors, collaborators (such as school administrators), reviewers, and publication editors to attend to them; developing and supporting appropriate research training; and attending to socioenvironmental aspects and data quality control elements of proposed research.

Identify minimum requirements for assessing the effectiveness of prevention strategies.

Evaluations of effectiveness must clearly specify and describe (directly or by reference to readily available supplementary sources or previous publications) each of the following elements and make provision for quantitative measurement of each of them:

- The components of the intervention strategy.
- Optimal and achieved levels of implementation of each component, from the perspective of both source and recipient.
- The prescribed and actual qualifications and training given to those implementing the strategy.
- The levels and types of community and organizational support for and opposition to the intervention.
- The character and extent of concurrent prevention activities in the research locale that affect the control and treatment subjects of the evaluation.
- The specific cognitive, affective, and behavioral measures used to assess outcomes.
- The characteristics of the treatment and the control populations under study (when present, whether randomly assigned or otherwise selected), including age, place of birth, sex, racial and ethnic identity, household structure and stability, household socioeconomic measures (household income and education level if available; other indicators such as residential density, vehicles owned, household furnishings), academic grades, block-level geographic information, drug experience, and previous exposure to or involvement in prevention activities.

Follow-up measures must be made at least 1 year after the initial intervention is completed, preferably at longer intervals when the expected rates of target behaviors to be affected are low or the sample size is small. Interim exposure to prevention curricula or other elements must be assessed.

Participant follow-up rates of 90 percent or greater are needed to measure accurately the effects on relatively uncommon outcomes such as regular cocaine use. In most cases this means that evaluation research designs must make provisions to retain identifiers of individual participants and locate them if necessary in environments discontinuous with the original site. An evaluation with a gross follow-up rate below 75 percent is of dubious validity to assess effects even on relatively common behaviors. Nonresponse analyses must be performed and reported.

A final note, which is not visible in the research under review and is not strictly necessary for effectiveness determination. We believe that the practical value of any evaluation is substantially improved if its performers take the trouble to give a careful accounting or best possible estimate of the unit costs of implementing the intervention, separately from the costs of the research components.

1

Illicit Drug Use
in the United States

The use of illegal drugs has been a long-standing problem in American society, a problem that has taken on a particular urgency in the last 30 years. In the early 1960s, a presidential commission stated: "The concern and the distress of the American people over the national problem of drug abuse is expressed every day in the newspapers, the magazines, scientific journals, public forums and in the home. It is a serious and many-faceted problem" (President's Advisory Commission on Narcotics and Drug Abuse, 1963:1). In 1971, President Nixon called drugs, especially heroin, America's public enemy number one. The 1980s saw the emergence of cocaine, particularly crack cocaine, as a new focus of concern. After President George Bush's televised address in September 1989 (his first as President) on a national drug control strategy, 64 percent of respondents to a *New York Times*-CBS poll rated drugs as the nation's number one problem (*New York Times*, 1990). Respondents to such surveys during that period typically rated crime and AIDS as the number two and number three problems—both of which are associated with drugs. As one measure of importance attached to this issue, in fiscal 1992 the federal government spent $12 billion on antidrug efforts, and state and local agencies together spent roughly the same amount (White House, 1992).

The rise and fall of public preoccupation with drugs correlate in complex ways with shifts in patterns and levels of drug use (Duster, 1970; Lidz and Walker, 1980; Courtwright, 1992). Perceptions about public issues are volatile, often affected by such factors as political campaigning, presidential initiatives, and competing dramatic events in the media (Rogers, 1983);

these, far more than the prosaic conditions of everyday life, determine the perception of "America's number one problem." Thus, by July 1990, less than a year after 64 percent of the public had rated drugs as the number one problem, only 10 percent rated it that high (*New York Times*, 1990). The subsequent focus on the war in the Persian Gulf, the disintegration of the Soviet empire, economic concerns, and presidential politics resulted in even lower rankings of the drug problem.

Students of public health are acutely aware that the premature mortality, epidemiologic sequelae, and economic costs of illness presently associated with alcohol or tobacco separately greatly outweigh the comparable measures for cocaine, heroin, and all other drugs combined (Harwood et al., 1984; Rice et al., 1990). But present hazards to public health are not necessarily the values lodged uppermost in the public account. Concerns about criminal enterprises and moral commitments, fear of an uncertain future, and promotions broadcast by industrial advertisers and political activists compete powerfully with clinical observations and epidemiologic estimates in guiding the hand of prevention research and practice.

Regardless of the priority that the public, political leaders, and the media attach to drug problems at particular points in time, drugs are unquestionably a significant social problem for the United States in the 1990s. Their significance is compounded by the fact that drug problems do not stand alone. They complicate—and are complicated by—other major concerns such as the rising costs of health care, the AIDS epidemic, racial divisions, and violent crime. It is beyond the scope of this report to deal with all the complexities of the drug problem; we take it as a cardinal point of reference, however, that issues of morality, health, crime, and economics are inextricably linked to both the perception and the reality of the problem. An analytical focus on drugs per se is a simplification necessary for clarity, brevity, and efficiency in the present task of informing the scientific agendas of research agencies specifically concerned with prevention.

In this introduction, we develop a profile of the drug problem, highlighting the known facts of greatest relevance to prevention research, as well as the gaps in knowledge that are most troubling. We begin with a discussion of how drug problems develop and how they are diagnosed in terms of individual impairment and community disturbance. We then describe the changing magnitude of such problems over the past 20 years during which relatively extensive data collection efforts have been undertaken; we point to such explanations for these trends as the relevant research permits. We then look at the distribution of drug problems across subgroups of the population in closer detail. The chapter concludes with recommendations concerning epidemiologic research that should improve the ability to follow trends in drug problems and to explain their dynamics in more certain and useful ways.

DIAGNOSING DRUG PROBLEMS

From a scientific perspective, two different but complementary ways to define, study, and respond to drug problems have evolved over the past 30 years. One way is grounded in the clinical (or individual) approach, diagnosing drug problems strictly as unhealthy conditions attaching to individuals, analogous to specific cases of an infectious or chronic disease. The other is an environmental (or community) approach, in which drug problems are viewed as disorders affecting social groups, such as the family, neighborhood, or society. Although both approaches are concerned with causes and consequences, such as family disruption and reduced life expectancy, the environmental approach is also concerned with social disturbance and polarization, labor market distortions, and the economic burden of illness. Individual drives and motives are more central to the clinical approach. The environmental view emphasizes broader influences on drug use behavior, for example, drug consumption motivated by economic gain among disadvantaged youth with limited opportunities.

The clinical and environmental models are closely related. The clinical model focuses on a subgroup of all drug users, those whose drug consumption is more advanced, deeply compulsive, poorly responsive to social or environmental changes, and (at least temporarily) very difficult for the individual to control. The environmental model views the majority of persons using illicit drugs as having motives to use them or to remain addicted that precede or go beyond psychological disorder. The social environment educes conformity to group norms and reactions to economic circumstances. When group norms and economic circumstances contribute to promoting drug use, individuals in that environment are more susceptible to exposure to and use of drugs.

The Individual Perspective

Clinical definitions of individual drug problems are based on a set of carefully enumerated criteria for assessing individual drug-consumption behavior and its physiological and functional consequences. The clinical approach is summarized in the concept of Psychoactive Substance Use Disorder, as defined in the *Diagnostic and Statistical Manual of Mental Disorders* (American Psychiatric Association, 1987), generally referred to as DSM-III-R. The DSM-III-R implicitly distinguishes three levels of drug-related behavior and functioning: *drug dependence*, the core disorder; *drug abuse*, a less severe disorder; and all other patterns, which fall below the threshold of clinical attention and are called *drug use*. A very similar classification and set of distinguishing criteria appear in the *International Statistical Classification of Diseases, Injuries, and Causes of Death* (World Health Organization, 1992).

It may be useful to envision these levels of drug-consumption behavior as a series of concentric circles: drug dependence at the center, a surrounding ring of abuse, a wide outer rim of use, and outside that the realm of *abstinence*. If we further envision the boundaries of the circles as flexible and porous, and if we map all of the population onto this landscape and observe things over time, we should not be surprised to see the size of the circles expand and contract as millions of individuals shift back and forth across the boundaries.

The specific drugs being consumed (whether heroin or cocaine, amphetamines or tranquilizers, even alcohol or cigarettes—which, although licit, can become clinically problematic) are not emphasized in the definition. After nearly a century of study and massive documentation of polydrug sequences and patterns, it is clear that many varieties of psychoactive substances can yield disorders of drug dependence or abuse (Levison et al., 1983; Jaffe, 1990). The particular physiological properties and psychological effects of specific drugs are not viewed as irrelevant but rather as one in a series of important factors. The dose taken, the route of administration (smoking, swallowing, snuffing, injecting), and the social environment can attenuate or exaggerate many of the behavioral differences that the chemicals induce.

The distinctions between the legal drugs—alcohol beverages and tobacco—and the illegal drugs— such as cocaine, marijuana, and heroin—are today much sharper in the law than in the eyes of the pharmacologists and epidemiologists who are counting deaths and illnesses and the clinicians who are helping people recover from dependence. Nevertheless, the focus in this report is on the patterns of consumption, the consequences, and the effects of preventive interventions against illegal drugs, which are the principal research concerns of the particular sponsors and immediate audience of this report.

Table 1.1 presents the clinical criteria delineated in the two diagnostic manuals cited above. For our purposes, *use*, *abuse*, and *dependence* can be characterized more simply as follows:

Dependence is characterized by high or frequent doses taken continuously over a period of at least one month; compulsion, craving, withdrawal symptoms, and/or severe consequences in terms of health or functional impairments are very likely to be experienced.

Abuse generally occurs at lower doses and/or frequencies than dependence, although levels of consumption may be sporadically heavy. There are some detectable adverse effects in terms of health or functioning, which may be quite serious or have serious consequences, such as injury and violence.

Drug use is defined as consumption of low and/or infrequent doses, sometimes called "experimental," "casual," or "social," such that damaging consequences are rare or minor.

TABLE 1.1 Correspondence Between the Criteria for Dependence[a] of the *International Statistical Classification of Diseases, Injuries, and Causes of Death* (10th rev.) (ICD-10) and the *Diagnostic and Statistical Manual of Mental Disorders* (3rd ed., rev.) DSM-III-R

ICD-10	DSM-III-R
Progressive neglect of alternative pleasures or interests in favor of substance use.	Important social, occupation, or recreational activities given up because of substance use.
Persisting with drug use despite clear evidence of overtly harmful consequences.	Continued substance use despite knowledge of having a persistent or recurrent social, psychological, or physical problem that is caused or exacerbated by the use of the substance.
Evidence of tolerance such that increased doses of the substance are required in order to achieve effects originally produced by lower doses.	Marked tolerance: need for markedly increased amounts of the substance in order to achieve intoxication or desired effect, or markedly diminished effect with continued use of the same amount.
Substance use with the intention of relieving withdrawal symptoms and subjective awareness that this strategy is effective.	Substance often taken to relieve or avoid withdrawal symptoms.
A physiological withdrawal state.	Characteristic withdrawal symptoms.
Strong desire or sense of compulsion to take drugs.	Persistent desire or one or more unsuccessful efforts to cut down or control substance use.
Evidence of an impaired capacity to control drug taking behavior in terms of its onset, termination or level of use.	Substance often taken in larger amounts or over a longer period than the person intended.
A narrowing of the personal repertoire of patterns of drug use, e.g., a tendency to drink alcoholic beverages in the same way on weekdays and weekends and whatever the social constraints regarding appropriate drinking behavior.	Frequent intoxication or withdrawal symptoms when expected to fulfill major role obligations at work, school, or at home or when substance use is physically hazardous.
Evidence that a return to substance use after a period of abstinence leads to a rapid reinstatement of other features of the syndrome than occurs with nondependent individuals.	A great deal of time spent in activities necessary to get the substance, taking the substance, or recovering from its effects.

[a]A dependence syndrome is present if three or more criteria are met (ICD: persistently) (DSM: continuously) in the previous month or (ICD: some time) (DSM: repeatedly) in the previous year.

SOURCES: World Health Organization (1992); American Psychiatric Organization (1987). Courtesy of Gerstein and Harwood (1990).

We must emphasize that, although drug use is not a clinical disorder, this does not imply that it is necessarily benign or trivial. It is reasonable to question whether any level of drug consumption should be counted as less than abuse for young adolescents. The *potential* for progression beyond use to abuse or dependence is always present, and the age of drug onset is related to the likelihood of continued and cumulative adverse effects. Those who initiate drug use at earlier ages are at greater risk of later abuse and dependence (Kandel et al., 1986).

The concepts of use, abuse, and dependence raise some important points that are discussed in the following sections: (1) age-related characteristics; (2) temporal sequence and progression; and (3) specific consequences associated with each stage.

Age-Related Characteristics

The onset or initiation of drug use has been studied in several cross-sectional and longitudinal investigations. The most important finding reveals that most experimentation with illicit drug use begins during adolescence. For some people, the initiation of cigarettes and alcohol (which are illicit for minors even though they are legal for adults to buy and use) begins even before the teenage years. Among the 12- to 17-year-old respondents to the 1990 National Household Survey on Drug Abuse who had ever used alcohol, the mean age of first use was 12.8; the corresponding figure for cigarettes was 11.5 (National Institute on Drug Abuse, 1991b). About one-fifth (21.0 percent) of the 12- to 13-year-old respondents had tried cigarettes, and one-fourth (25.9 percent) had tried alcohol. In a state-wide survey of New York students, 5 percent of the students age 12 or younger were classified as "heavy" drinkers according to criteria developed for adolescents—that is, they drank at least once a week and drank relatively large amounts on a typical drinking occasion (Barnes and Welte, 1987). Some marijuana use also occurs among preteens. In the 1990 Household Survey, 2.9 percent of the 12- to 13-year-old respondents had tried marijuana (National Institute on Drug Abuse, 1991b). These findings are consistent with those of Kandel and Logan (1984): the rate of initiation for drug use increases around age 10, with one-fifth of the cohort reporting ever using alcohol before age 10. The average age of initiation for cigarette and marijuana use is 12 and 13.

Relatively few people begin using drugs—or even any particular type of drug, unless it was never previously available—after reaching 21-25 years of age, except for prescription drugs. The risk for initiation of cigarette, alcohol, and marijuana use subsides for the majority of youth by age 20, and for illicit drugs other than cocaine by age 21 (Kandel and Logan, 1984). The implication for prevention is that efforts to prevent the onset of most drug use probably should concentrate on the age group just entering adolescence, if not those younger. Most current interventions have acknowledged this implication. More effective interventions for older adolescents or adults who have already initiated consumption could focus not on preventing onset—apart from cocaine use—but on encouraging cessation and on forestalling the intensification of drug use to the point of abuse and dependence. We should note that, in addition to these patterns of early onset of illicit drug use, a distinct problem has developed in the elderly with abuse of prescribed drugs. However, there is little theoretical work or intervention research on this problem, and it is so different from the topics treated here that we must defer it to later assessment in another study.

Sequence and Progression of Drug Involvement

Populations of young people in the United States and other industrialized countries show a remarkable degree of uniformity, dating back to surveys in the early 1970s, in the sequence of their drug involvement. Research findings reveal that young people who have used multiple drugs appear to do so by progressing systematically through a sequence of stages. Drug abuse also develops through a specific sequence of increasing drug involvement.

Hamburg et al. (1975) found that adolescents tended to experiment first with coffee and tea; this was followed sequentially by use of wine and beer, tobacco, hard liquor, marijuana, hallucinogens, stimulants and depressants, and narcotics. The onset of each of these substances was separate, with relatively few adolescents progressing through the hierarchy without using each of the preceding drugs. Similar results were found during the same period on a larger sample by Kandel (1975). The most frequently documented sequence involves four stages of onset:

1. beer or wine,
2. tobacco and/or liquor,
3. marijuana, and
4. "hard" drugs such as sedatives, tranquilizers, or cocaine.

This pattern does not suggest that everyone moves from (1) all the way through (4). However, for those who do, the nature of movement is restricted and cumulative—somewhat like a series of gates through which one can pass only in a specific order. For this reason, the term *gateway drugs* is used to refer to the first and second stages.

It is typical to find that 80 percent of a sample (see Kandel, 1975; O'Donnell et al., 1976; Clayton and Voss, 1981; Clayton et al., 1987), to the degree that they reported any drug use, did so in conformity with the order indicated above and not in some other sequence, and that those who departed from this sequence did so minimally, most commonly by using cigarettes prior to any alcohol. Rarely does someone use cocaine without previously using the drugs in the prior stages; in fact, Kandel and others (Yamaguchi and Kandel, 1984a, 1984b; O'Donnell and Clayton, 1982; Henningfield et al., 1990) have shown that use of marijuana is virtually a necessary condition for cocaine use in youth.

Contrary to prevailing findings, Newcomb and Bentler (1986) concluded that alcohol was not the major gateway drug. In their Los Angeles sample, alcohol use was fairly stable, with little cross-influence on other drugs. Cigarettes, in contrast, were identified as the gateway drug facilitating progression to marijuana and harder drug use, particularly for earlier ages. Rather than viewing the initiation and progression of drug use as a single general sequence, they suggested several smaller sequences, and that at higher levels of drug involvement, the use of cigarettes, marijuana, and hard drugs have a synergistic or reciprocal effect of increasing drug involvement. In a similar vein, Yamaguchi and Kandel (1984a) have suggested that between marijuana and all other illicit drugs may come a specific stage of using prescription-type pills, especially tranquilizers, while Donovan and Jessor (1985) have suggested that "problem drinking" (alcohol abuse) is a separate stage after marijuana and before other drugs.

The later-stage drugs, which are distinguished here as illicit drugs (prohibited for adults as well as minors), are added onto, rather than replacing, the earlier drugs. The number of times the earlier-sequence drugs are consumed is a sensitive indicator; in most studies the likelihood of moving to a further stage increases the more intensively and continuously the earlier-initiated drugs are consumed. In this sense the sequence not only is ordered in time but also has scalar properties, which make the level of each category predictive of the next. For example, the more extensive or intensive the use of marijuana, the greater the likelihood of trying cocaine. Among 12- to 17-year-old respondents to the 1990 National Household Survey on Drug Abuse (1991b), of those who had consumed marijuana in the month preceding the interview (one-twentieth of the sample), 37.0 percent had used drugs other than marijuana in the past month, including 9.8 percent reporting past-month cocaine use; of the remaining vast majority, who had no past-month marijuana consumption, 3.1 percent had used other drugs and less than 0.5 percent (the lower limit of statistical detection) reported cocaine use (Table 1.2).

The sequential character is unlikely to be pharmacological in origin, but rather economical and sociological—that is, alcohol and tobacco are inexpensive and very widely accessible to young people because they are legally mass-marketed to adults; marijuana in turn has preceded other drugs in part because it is generally less expensive and more widely available than cocaine, pills, or heroin and in part because it is viewed as less dangerous.

TABLE 1.2 Percentage Reporting Use of Selected Drugs in the Past Month, by Age Group and Marijuana Use in the Past Month, 1990

Age Group and Drugs Used in the Past Month	Marijuana Use in the Past Month		Total
	No	Yes	
Total	(N = 8,644)	(N = 615)	(N = 9,259)
Alcohol	49.0	90.8	51.2
Cigarettes	24.9	59.7	26.7
Drugs other than marijuana	1.4	23.8	2.6
Nonmedical use of any			
psychotherapeutics[a]	1.0	10.0	1.4
Cocaine	0.2	11.2	0.8
12-17 Years Old	(N = 2,085)	(N = 92)	(N = 2,177)
Alcohol	20.9	91.6	24.5
Cigarettes	8.6	67.3	11.6
Drugs other than marijuana	3.1	37.0	4.9
Nonmedical use of any			
psychotherapeutics	1.9	17.6	2.7
Cocaine	b	9.8	0.6
18-25 Years Old	(N = 1,812)	(N = 240)	(N = 2,052)
Alcohol	58.9	93.1	63.3
Cigarettes	27.5	59.0	31.5
Drugs other than marijuana	2.5	27.8	5.7
Nonmedical use of any			
psychotherapeutics	1.3	11.4	2.6
Cocaine	0.8	11.4	2.2
26-34 Years Old	(N = 2,139)	(N = 216)	(N = 2,355)
Alcohol	60.9	89.5	63.3
Cigarettes	34.7	66.9	37.5
Drugs other than marijuana	1.3	23.6	3.2
Nonmedical use of any			
psychotherapeutics	0.7	10.6	1.6
Cocaine	0.5	14.7	1.7
35 Years and Older	(N = 2,608)	(N = 67)	(N = 2,675)
Alcohol	47.8	88.3	48.6
Cigarettes	23.9	46.1	24.3
Drugs other than marijuana	1.0	10.6	1.1
Nonmedical use of any			
psychotherapeutics	0.8	b	0.8
Cocaine	b	6.3	0.2

[a]Nonmedical use of any prescription-type stimulant, sedative, tranquilizer, or analgesic; does not include over-the-counter drugs.

[b]Low precision; no estimate reported.

SOURCE: National Institute on Drug Abuse (1991b:Table 3.8).

The tendency for heavier use of earlier drugs to correlate with greater likelihood of using later ones is also, to a certain degree, sociological in nature: more intensive users tend to segregate themselves and be segregated by others, increasing their exposure to diversified drug sellers and consumers. There may also be a pharmacological component as individuals begin to take one drug to modify the effects of others (Johnston and O'Malley, 1986), e.g., taking cocaine to counter alcohol-induced drowsiness or taking heroin to take the edge off cocaine.

Consumption of one or more of these substances may progress from use to abuse and further to dependence. The timing and nature of such transitions (which are probabilistic rather than ironclad or deterministic in nature) vary with individual factors, by substance, and by mode of administration (for example, snorting cocaine versus smoking it, or injecting it in combination with other drugs such as heroin). It is critical to note that progression occurs in a minority of cases. Just as most alcohol users do not become dependent, most individuals who try illicit drugs do not progress beyond use; they remain at a low level or move back to abstinence (Johnston et al., 1991a).

Perhaps the drug with the highest proportion of continuation of use beyond experimentation or occasional use is tobacco: after as few as two cigarettes smoked, one-third or more continue to use for a considerable length of time (Henningfield, 1984). While two-thirds of high school seniors reported ever trying a cigarette, 29 percent reported use in the last month. Cigarettes were used daily by more of the respondents (18 percent) than any other drug. The high rates of continuation for cigarette smoking are exceeded by occasional heavy drinking defined as the consumption of 5 or more drinks at least once in the last 2 weeks. Over one-third (35 percent) of the high school sample and a young adult sample engaged in occasional heavy drinking.

Even in the case of a drug with as fearsome a popular reputation for inducing dependence as cocaine, most users do not progress to the point of dependence. It is sensible, then, to consider that every transition—nonuse to use, use to abuse, abuse to dependence—is an opportunity for preventive factors to operate, which both encourages and complicates the task of designing preventive interventions and measuring their effects.

Consequences

The consequences of drug consumption vary in severity, type, and how rapidly they become manifest. The occurrence and severity of most consequences are correlated either with the level of current consumption or the cumulative level of consumption for many years beyond onset. The most well-known consequences include acute health crises such as overdose death or traumatic injuries while intoxicated (Simons-Morton et al., 1989); chronic or cumulative damages such as tissue deterioration, scarring, and oncogenesis (in smokers' throats and lungs, smokeless tobacco users' oral membranes, drinkers' livers, sniffers' nasal membranes, intravenous injectors' veins); a variety of endocrine, neurological, and central nervous system degradation, some reversible and some irreversible (see Spencer and Boren, 1990); AIDS (Feucht et al., 1990; Chitwood et al., 1990); criminality (Faupel, 1988; Dembo et al., 1991); and developmental disability (Block et al., 1990; Nathan, 1990). Because the population has many more users than abusers or those who are dependent, there are large numbers of people who are individually at some small degree of risk for impairment, and small numbers of people are at high risk of consequences. No quantitative analysis at this time indicates how these total group risks compare in size with each other. But if we work by analogy from the analyses of population risks for cancer and cardiovascular disease, we may assume that the severity of risks are distributed log-normally—which means that each level of risk is multiplied by some factor of the former, not merely added to it. This argues for approaches to prevention that seek to reduce risk factors in both the high-risk minority and the middle majority of the distribution curve (see the appendix).

Perhaps the most critical feature of youthful drug use is the potential for interfering with normal biological, psychological, and social development. Youngsters who become involved with drugs beyond experimental use are at greater risk of failing to accomplish necessary educational and developmental tasks. This is not necessarily an objective of drug use by youth, which is generally functional and goal-oriented (Jessor, 1983). They use drugs variously as a way to experience pleasure or risk, gain acceptance by a peer group, assert authority and independence, reject conventional institutions of society, assert important characteristics of their identity, or mark the transition to adulthood (Jessor, 1983; Johnston and O'Malley, 1986; Murray and Perry, 1984). These motivations for drug use are characteristic of normal psychosocial development and do not differ from the goals associated with behaviors not related to drug use (Jessor, 1991). The underlying motivations for drug use are not static but vary by drug, and further by the degree of drug involvement (Johnston and O'Malley, 1986). For example, smoking onset is strongly related to social factors in early adolescence but shifts to internal motivations by late adolescence (Pederson and Lefcoe, 1985).

Despite these normalizing aspects, drug use jeopardizes the normal processes of development. The use of one or more classes of drugs between adolescence and young adulthood has been found to interfere with normal development by compromising physical and psychological health, the performance of traditional work and family roles, and the level of education achieved in young adulthood (Kandel et al., 1986). Developmental disability tends to be a condition that is difficult to correct or to compensate for adequately in later life.

The Community Perspective

In addition to the individual perspective, which is characteristic of the clinical model, drug problems can be viewed from a socioenvironmental perspective. The disciplines of epidemiology and public health, for example, introduce the triad of the host (the individual who is a potential or current drug consumer), the agent (specific drug varieties), and environmental structures and processes that may bring hosts and agents together or keep them apart (Duncan, 1988; Last and Wallace, 1991). This framework was applied by the Institute of Medicine (1989) Panel on Opportunities for Research on Prevention of Alcohol Problems; it is addressed more extensively in Chapter 2 and in the appendix. Its models of drug-taking are psychosocial, emphasizing how an individual behaves in the context of different social groups (family, peers, markets, other social institutions) (Akers et al., 1979), and cultural, emphasizing ideas, beliefs, and values that tend to be associated with ethnic, socioeconomic, and geographic populations (Buchanan, 1991, 1992).

The major societal factors of concern include the existence of residential blocks that are overrun by drug markets and mass media that have glamorized drug taking. Individuals in high-exposure environments may become involved with drugs in entirely different ways and for different reasons than individuals elsewhere. An otherwise relatively low-risk individual coming of age in such a high-exposure environment has different prospects than does a low-exposure individual in a low-exposure environment, that is, one in which drugs are marginal and nearly invisible. For young people in such areas, the attractiveness of the income and the job opportunities associated with drug trafficking versus other kinds of income-producing jobs may be substantial. The exposure level to drug-related consequences such as violent trauma, unemployment, and AIDS may be high even for nonusers.

TRENDS IN DRUG USE

The overall epidemiology of drug consumption—that is, patterns of use of drugs in populations—has been monitored on a national basis principally through two surveys regularly sponsored by the National Institute on Drug Abuse (NIDA): the National Household Survey on Drug Abuse (NIDA, 1991a,b), which has been administered periodically since 1972, and the annual (since 1975) High School Senior Survey (Johnston et al., 1991a,b).

In addition, various efforts to monitor specific consequences associated with drug use, abuse, and dependence have been mounted, providing for analyses over time. The most long-standing and methodologically consistent of these data series is the Drug Abuse Warning Network (DAWN) system, which collects data on emergency room episodes involving drug use in a national sample of emergency rooms and medical examiner reports of drug-related fatalities in more than a dozen major metropolitan areas. (We note, however, that the validity of DAWN data are subject to troubling quality control problems in the data collection process, first noted in a methodological report to the Drug Enforcement Administration by the Franklin Research Institute in 1978 and never adequately resolved. These results should be interpreted with due consideration to the methodological constraints.) The Drug Use Forecasting (DUF) system collects urine specimens and interview data from a sample of arrestees in about two dozen major municipal police departments.

In addition, reports on treatment episodes are collected from a limited number of states that voluntarily continue the Client Oriented Data Acquisition Process (CODAP), a federal system that was established in 1972 but for which federal support was discontinued after 1980. A new system of collecting annual statistical information on the treatment of people with substance abuse problems in the United States, the Client Data System, is being formed in response to legislation included in the Anti-Drug Abuse Act of 1988 (Blanken, 1989). Several of these data series are examined on a regular basis by the Community Epidemiology Working Group, comprised of representatives from 26 metropolitan areas.

More localized trend data are rare and not so continuous over time; for example, New York State data for schoolchildren were collected in 1973, 1978, 1983, and 1989-1990 (Puccio and Simeone, 1991; Barnes and Welte, 1987; Kandel et al., 1976). The Substance Abuse and Mental Health Services Administration has recently begun to stimulate and support state-level household surveys and other data collection as part of treatment evaluation and assessment activities.

In recent years, results from the two broad types of data collection systems—data from surveys of probability samples of individuals and data collected from case contacts in clinical or criminal justice settings—have been somewhat divergent, creating challenges in assessing the meaning of statistical trends in drug consumption and associated problems.

Population Survey Results

The household and high school senior surveys showed considerable declines in current illicit drug use (that is, any use within the 30 days preceding the survey) in the 1980s (Figure 1.1). Among high school seniors

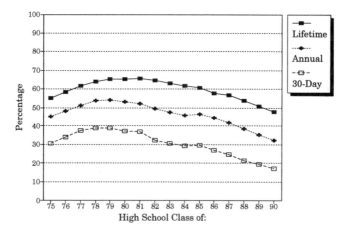

FIGURE 1.1 Index of Illicit Drugs: Lifetime, Annual, and 30-Day Prevalence, 1975-1990. SOURCE: Johnston et al. (1991a).

in the graduating class of 1989, about one-fifth (20 percent) reported having taken an illicit drug at least once in the past 30 days; this figure is about half what it was 10 years earlier among the class of 1979 (39 percent). Marijuana, the most widely used illicit drug, accounts for much of the overall change, falling continuously since 1979 (Figure 1.2). Consumption patterns characteristic of abuse and dependence have declined even more sharply among seniors. More than one-tenth of the class of 1979 reported smoking marijuana on a daily (or near daily) basis, compared with less than 3 percent of the class of 1989.

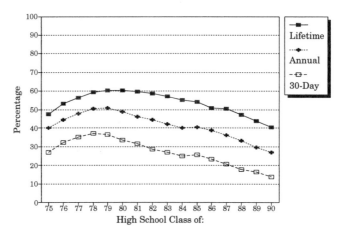

FIGURE 1.2 Marijuana: Lifetime, Annual, and 30-Day Prevalence, 1975-1990. SOURCE: Johnston et al. (1991a).

The pattern of cocaine use is more complicated. Figure 1.3 shows that it increased sharply between 1976 and 1980, then increased slightly more through 1986, a year that saw the highly publicized deaths from cocaine overdose of two nationally known young athletes; after 1986 cocaine use fell sharply. Public concern, in contrast, increased dramatically from 1986 to 1989, at just about the same time that survey measures of student consumption were beginning to decline.

College students are surveyed annually in conjunction with the surveys of high school seniors. The decline in illicit drugs evident among high school students also occurred among college students: a college student in 1989 was about half as likely to use illicit drugs, compared with 1980. Current marijuana use was 16 percent in 1989 compared with 34 percent in 1980, and current cocaine use was down to 2.8 percent from 7 percent. Similar declines were reflected in the household surveys. Consumption of illicit drugs is most prevalent among young adults ages 18-25 and older. Current marijuana use for this group was 35 percent in 1979, and less than half that in 1988 (16 percent). Similarly, current cocaine use dropped by half, from 9.3 percent to 4.5 percent.

It is clear from survey data that the overall profile of household and student population involvement with illicit drugs is down—and down dramatically (see Figure 1.4). How these trends translate into higher levels of consumption is less certain. The 1990 National Household Survey reported that, among those who used cocaine at all in the last year, 10 percent used the drug once a week or more, and 4 percent used it daily or almost daily; among the 1985 past-year users, 5 percent were weekly users and 2 percent

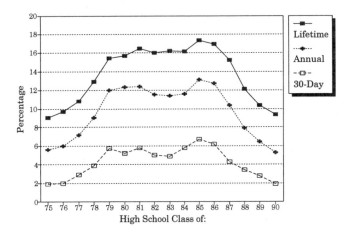

FIGURE 1.3 Cocaine: Lifetime, Annual, and 30-Day Prevalence, 1975-1990. SOURCE: Johnston et al. (1991a).

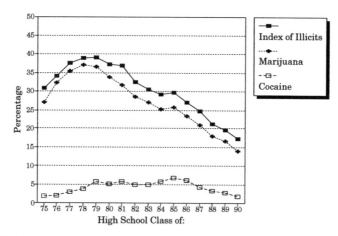

FIGURE 1.4 Illicit Drug Index, Marijuana, Cocaine: 30-Day Prevalences, 1975-1990. SOURCE: Johnston et al. (1991a).

daily or almost daily users. The surveys of high school seniors showed contrasting findings: in 1991, 1.4 percent of high school seniors who used in the past month were daily or almost daily users; in 1990, the corresponding figure was 1.9 percent; in 1989, 2.8 percent.

Thus, even among the general populations covered by these two surveys, there is some question about the degree to which drug involvement at the level of abuse and dependence may be declining, despite the overall drop in rates of use. Moreover, there are some very significant gaps in the population covered by the two surveys, and the poorly represented populations may be behaving differently from those who are well represented. The high school senior surveys, for example, do not include high school dropouts, and there is ample evidence that drug problems are likely to be more severe among segments of the population in which dropout rates are likely to be greatest, such as economically disadvantaged populations in inner cities. The household surveys also exclude all individuals not living in conventional households, such as those in group quarters, institutions, or transient places. Both surveys rely on individuals voluntarily agreeing to participate in the study; people who are having severe drug problems are undoubtedly less likely to be available and agreeable to participate in a lengthy interview than are unimpaired household members.

Validity and Reliability of Survey Data

Any data collection system that relies on self-reports must address the issue of validity—do people tell the truth (or know the truth) when they are asked to tell a stranger about their own (or another's) use of illegal drugs? A variety of studies have been undertaken to establish the validity of such surveys (Rouse et al., 1985). Perhaps the most general conclusion that can be supported is that most people are willing to be reasonably truthful (within the bounds of their capability) under the proper conditions.

"The proper conditions," of course, is the key phrase. Evidence from other areas of survey research suggests that, when respondents believe they are guaranteed anonymity and confidentiality, when they accept the scientific or practical value of the survey, when they accept the legitimacy of the survey, then they tend to be generally truthful (Forman and Linney, 1991; Rouse et al., 1985; Murray and Perry, 1987). Whether these conditions are met in the household drug use survey, the school-based surveys of students, or the mail-out questionnaire follow-up surveys of high school graduates is debatable. The survey operators have worked to develop methods of shielding answers and reassuring respondents, and the federal government has enacted legislation to protect the confidentiality of individual data. The degree to which confidentiality assurances are believed may vary with social or cultural affiliations and personality characteristics of the respondents. Some of these differences are correlates and predictors of risk for drug use (Moncher et al., 1991). Some youth at high risk for drug use may not divulge any illicit drug use if they suspect the interviewer knows who they are for fear of apprehension by legal authorities or punishment by some other social system such as social welfare or education.

But even if the precision and validity of the survey are somewhat compromised by biases, other tests suggest the reliability of trend data over time. One such factor is the presumption of constancy of bias; even if individual prevalence estimates are systematically biased downward by underreporting, so long as the bias is relatively constant from year to year, trend estimates may be quite reliable. This presumption is supported by the fact that other responses to drug consumption questions have not drifted away from the self-report trend, as might occur if individuals were becoming increasingly reluctant to self-report. For example, the high school seniors survey asks respondents what proportion of their friends use a given drug. Even if there were a change in willingness to report self-behaviors, there should be somewhat less change in willingness to report unnamed friends' behaviors. However, seniors' reports of their friends' drug practices parallel very closely the trend in reports of their own use.

A second methodological support for validity is that different drugs display different trends over time; self-reported marijuana use declined earlier than did cocaine, and reported use of other drugs (including alcohol) has not declined. A third type of evidence bearing on trend validity is that different self-report methods produce similar trend results. Self-administered mail-out questionnaires, group-administered school-based questionnaires, and household interviews using self-completed, sealed answer sheets all provide similar trends. A fourth indication of validity is that the absolute levels of reported drug involvement are substantial; large numbers of respondents do freely admit to experiences with illicit drugs; lifetime marijuana prevalence among some age groups is well over 50 percent, demonstrating that most users do indeed admit to this on a self-report basis.

Finally, the data show convergent and predictive validity. That is, reported levels of consumption relate to other variables in ways that seem internally consistent: more use among males, more use among individuals who are otherwise delinquent and less academically successful, less use among married persons and pregnant women. Crider (1985) compared trends in indicators of heroin epidemics (hepatitis-B, heroin-related emergency room visits, heroin-related deaths, and average retail heroin purity) with trends based on self-report data from the National Household Surveys. She found that the trends in indicators were consistent with the household data. And yet there is some evidence to suggest that not all the survey methods are equally accurate. For example, telephone procedures (McAuliffe et al., 1991) may be problematic with younger respondents (Frank, 1985) or with some ethnic groups (Aquilino and Losciuto, 1990). And some researchers have suggested that physiological test procedures are useful in increasing the validity of self-reports of cigarette smoking among younger students— although not among older students (Werch et al., 1987).

It would be useful to employ methods other than traditional self-report, and a number of alternative (or supplementary) techniques have been attempted, including randomized response (Warner, 1965), bogus pipeline (Murray and Perry, 1987), nomination technique (Sirken, 1975), and item-count method (Miller, 1985). A number of studies have been devoted to ascertaining the conditions under which respondents tend to be truthful (Forman and Linney, 1991), and this remains a very active arena for research. Increasing the use of biological validation techniques (urine samples, saliva samples, hair samples, breath tests) is likely to lead to better methods of objective validation. The difference in self-reported rates of smoking may be confounded by age and experience. The bogus pipeline, in which respondents are asked to provide a saliva sample only to give the appearance that their verbal reports will be validated by chemical tests for traces of cigarette smoking, was found to increase reporting of drug use by younger people, but only the first time they were surveyed (Murray and Perry, 1987). Physical measures tend to be better indicators of recent heavy use, but they are less sensitive to sporadic or light use. So, for various reasons, the traditional self-report method under the proper conditions continues to be the most practical.

There is a critical need to reinvigorate methodological studies of the validity of standard measures, to reconfirm that some critical findings about validity and reliability from studies in the 1970s remain applicable. The drug literature needs to be compared with methodological work on validation of self-report methods involving other sensitive subjects, such as sexual behavior, criminal activities, and compliance with medical regimens. Biases in self-reporting need to be reassessed and methodological investigation needs to be supported concerning the differences among results from general population studies, case observations in criminal justice and clinical settings, and ethnographic investigations.

Aside from problems of validity, survey data are subject to nonresponse error due to incomplete population coverage and insufficient response rates. Here, too, an important consideration is consistency over time. If response rates or coverage were to change from year to year, that could produce spurious changes in apparent prevalence results. Clearly, the surveys do not cover all the affected populations equally well, and they undoubtedly underestimate the number of people involved with drugs at any one point in time. The household and the high school senior survey results seem to accurately represent overall trends in drug use in the general population, but not necessarily in the highest risk groups. This fact limits what the committee can conclude from existing trend data in its generalizability to the highest-risk populations, especially school dropouts, those who are unemployed and do not have permanent addresses, and those engaged in illegal activities.

Youth at the greatest risk for drug use are those more likely to be absent from school and to cut classes (see Hawkins et al., 1987). The absence of this high-risk group from the present surveys imposes a limitation on interpretation of the drug estimates. Research has established higher rates of alcohol and drug use among street kids (McKirnan and Johnston, 1986): 65 percent of street youth were identified as moderate-heavy and heavy drinkers of alcohol, and 23 percent of the sample as almost daily users of marijuana.

DAWN Data

The Drug Abuse Warning Network (DAWN) data, unlike the survey data, showed dramatic increases between 1985 and 1989 in emergency room cases linked to cocaine (Table 1.3). Since 1989, there has been a rough leveling off or slight to substantial decline in emergency room cocaine incidents in the DAWN cities under NIDA's community epidemiology research program, although quarter-to-quarter trends have fluctuated quite dramatically in both directions, presumably reflecting instabilities in the cocaine market or, possibly, endemic quality control problems in emergency room data collection (Community Epidemiology Working Group, 1992a,b). This probably reflects the overrepresentation of minorities and other high-risk groups in treatment populations, especially in emergency rooms. Not until the last quarter of 1989 was there a downturn in this indicator of

TABLE 1.3   ER Cocaine Mentions (cocaine noted in medical record)

	1985	1986	1987	1988	1989
Total Cocaine Mentions:	10,248	18,579	32,052	42,512	42,145
Number Injecting Cocaine:	3,911	5,460	9,041	11,471	9,346

SOURCES: Adams et al. (1990).

problems associated with cocaine abuse, although the medical examiner data showed some evidence of reaching a peak as early as the last quarter of 1988. The seeming divergence between the two systems in trends related to cocaine (the household and high school senior surveys showing declines from 1985-1991 when the DAWN data showed increases) is perhaps due to their differing sensitivities to use versus abuse and dependence. Individuals who report use at a given point in time may escalate to abuse or dependence after an interval of several years, so that changes in abuse and dependence indicators may lag behind shifts in the onset of use by several years. Thus the increased use rates observed in surveys through the mid-1980s would not be expected to result in a peaking of the medical problems typical of dependence until the late 1980s.

The decline observed in the last quarter of 1989 is consistent with the peak-lag hypothesis. Data from the first quarter of 1990 continue the decline (Adams, 1990). The fact that there was essentially a flattening prior to the decline lends further credence to the belief that cocaine problems are receding in the wake (several years after) of the general recession in use. However, it is equally plausible that the patterns of abuse and dependence tapped by DAWN are decoupled from the general population trends, representing population subgroups whose drug involvement has not changed in the same way that the general population has.

Data on Treatment Demand

Although treatment data have not been collected systematically enough during the 1980s to make clear statements about trends (see Gerstein and Harwood, 1990), there is little doubt that demand for treatment, particularly for cocaine abuse, increased during the latter 1980s, as use prevalence statistics declined. As with the DAWN data, one likely explanation has to do with the time lag between the onset of use and the development of dependence; the alternative explanation is that treatment populations are distinct from the general population.

Another problem associated with drug consumption is the delayed effect of perinatal exposure, especially to crack cocaine. More pregnant women are said to be using crack cocaine in particular, and some hospitals have reported high proportions of drug-exposed newborns (Chasnoff, 1989; Chasnoff et al., 1989, 1990). Whether the proportions of affected newborns are currently increasing or decreasing is hard to know, although the absolute levels are clearly unacceptably high. "Crack babies" are believed to have specific affective, cognitive, and behavioral problems (Chavez et al., 1989; Kusserow, 1990; Zuckerman et al., 1989; LeBlanc et al., 1987). Some school systems are now developing training programs to help teachers deal with the influx of such children into the education system (Barth, 1991). It is difficult to ascertain the extent to which the problems of crack babies are due to drug effects as such rather than other negative exposures in the child's environment such as poor hygiene, poor nutrition, lack of medical care, haphazard and neglectful parenting, etc.

Moreover, there is a "bias against the null hypothesis"; that is, the tendency for journals to publish results from studies that show effects more often than studies that fail to show effects (Koren et al., 1989). Nevertheless, it is clear that widespread crack consumption among young, economically disadvantaged women has substantially exacerbated the problem of perinatal exposure to illicit drugs. It has also substantially removed the earlier neonatal advantage associated with lower marijuana use by young black than by young white women.

Drug Abuse and AIDS

One of the most dramatic consequences of drug abuse and dependence is the high probability of contracting acquired immune deficiency syndrome (AIDS). As of March 1990, 28 percent of all persons (N = 126,127) diagnosed with AIDS were infected with the human immunodeficiency virus (HIV) by intravenous drug use—of those, heterosexuals were 21 percent and homosexual/bisexual males were another 7 percent. Fifty percent of all women diagnosed with AIDS were infected through intravenous drug use (Centers for Disease Control, 1990). Sharing HIV-contaminated needles is the way in which this infection has spread. AIDS is thought to be transmitted by small amounts of blood contained in needles, syringes, or bottle cap "cookers" shared among drug users (Friedman and Klein, 1987). The rates of needle sharing are high. One study found that 70 percent of intravenous drug users shared needles with others, and 86 percent had shared a cooker (Booth et al., 1991). Intravenous drug users do not use condoms regularly, placing their partners at high risk for contracting AIDS through sexual contact (Feucht et al., 1990). As many as two-thirds of this high-risk group have never used a condom (Booth et al., 1991). Although each estimate of the number of intravenous drug users has a fairly wide confidence interval (Spencer, 1989), a number of estimates converge on a figure of approximately 1.1 million intravenous drug users in the United States (Turner et al., 1989). Approximately 25 percent of them are HIV infected (Centers for Disease Control, 1987). Most are heterosexual and sexually active.

A second group that runs a very high risk of becoming infected with AIDS are crack cocaine users who exchange sex for drugs (Fullilove and Fullilove, 1989). As a drug, crack cocaine does not necessarily dispose users to heightened sexuality. But the way in which this drug is marketed has fatal long-term consequences. Many women who have become dependent on the trade of sex for drugs, and many young male sellers receive payment in sexual favors. Among a sample of black adolescent crack users, 25 percent reported the exchange of sex for drugs or money, the rates being similar for both males and females. One study found the rate of exchange of sex for drugs or money to be higher among females than males (Feucht et al., 1990). Only 26 percent of males and 18 percent of females had used a condom in their last sexual encounter, and over one-third of males and over one-half of females reported a history of sexually transmitted diseases. As a consequence, these drug users have high rates of sexually transmitted diseases and are one of the largest new AIDS high-risk groups (Jonsen, 1993). Data are not yet available on the rate of HIV infection among crack cocaine users. Since most are heterosexual and sexually active, they constitute a major group through which the AIDS virus can move into the general, heterosexual population (Centers for Disease Control, 1987). Of women admitted to a New York City hospital with pelvic inflammatory disease, 87 percent of those found HIV positive were crack users (Hoegsberg et al., 1989). Compared with nonusers, women who used crack had twice as many sexual partners per month.

Criminal Justice Statistics

Another indicator of problems with drug use in general, and cocaine use more specifically, comes from the criminal justice system. Here too, there appears to be some divergence from general downward trends in prevalence and specific problem indicators: murders and other violence related to drug trafficking seems to have increased in the nation's larger cities and other cities as well. Compared with data from population surveys, the criminal justice data on drug-related crimes are less systematically obtained (because of the difficulty in determining the degree to which drugs are involved), and they overrepresent high-risk groups, yet there can be little doubt that there is an enormous problem in some parts of our larger cities. Whether the problem is growing or expanding to other areas is less clear.

One new source of data on drug use is the National Institute of Justice's

Drug Use Forecasting (DUF) system, which is a program that obtains information on drug use by recent arrestees via interviews and urinalysis. Data from this system show that a very high proportion of arrestees in cities around the country test positive for drug use. The figures for cocaine in particular are dramatic, with an average of nearly 50 percent of recent arrestees in the DUF sample testing positive (which indicates that cocaine was used within 48-72 hours of arrest) (O'Neil and Visher, 1992).

Trends are more problematic to assess for technical reasons—because of the nonprobability nature of the samples, changes over time in coverage, differences in procedures, etc.—but, except for those in Washington, D.C., there does not appear to be any recent clear downturn in the proportions of arrestees who are testing positive.

Reasons for the Decline in the General Population

The evidence for a decline in illicit drug consumption among the general population is fairly compelling; a natural question is why the decline has occurred. The evidence from the high school senior surveys is that, for both marijuana and cocaine, as the perceived risk of harm and perceived normative impropriety of these drugs increased, consumption rates decreased. At the same time there was no decline in the perceived availability of either drug. Dramatic, highly publicized incidents in the case of cocaine might well account for the rapidity of the shift in health beliefs and social norms about cocaine. There were no such dramatic events in the case of marijuana, but beliefs about that drug shifted anyway, more gradually but quite decisively, presumably as a consequence of an accretion of factors.

For example, one might hypothesize a self-correcting process of social cognition, by which information about the bad consequences of long-term heavy use feeds back over time from older to younger cohorts, suppressing the onset of a behavior pattern that had been premised on more benign, less accurate beliefs about chronic drug effects (Feldman, 1968; Musto, 1987; Siegel, 1992). Or the process may involve an ebb and flow of normative approval based on slowly turning tides of generational values and experience. Or the resistance of young people to starting drug experimentation may have increased as a result of widely diffused primary prevention efforts in the schools and mass media. We cannot readily separate the perceptions of hazard and the social norms associated with marijuana or cocaine, so closely are these two elements correlated in the survey data (Johnston et al., 1991a,b).

The evidence clearly demonstrates a decline in illicit drug use among the general population, and there may also be a recent time-lagged decline in most indicators of dependence and abuse in the general population. But not all dependence and abuse indicators are declining. Criminal justice system data in particular and some of the survey data on consumption levels are not encouraging. Plausible reasons for disparity in trends include the time-lag hypothesis: that drug abuse or dependence emerges in large part within relatively limited subgroups of the population, and that the rates of onset of drug use in these subgroups are not changing in step with the bulk of the population. Alternatively, or in addition, the lack of correspondence between criminal justice system data and indicators of dependence and abuse may be influenced by the increasing attention of the public and government to drugs, which might also increase the sensitivity of emergency room staff to drug-related cases.

To sort out these explanations, it is necessary to look at more detailed characteristics than broad national aggregates. National statistics are not designed to represent any particular community. Just as economic booms and busts are not uniformly distributed throughout the country, drug consumption is by no means uniformly distributed. To understand a particular community's drug problem in detail, it is necessary to gather more detailed information specific to that community, recognizing that an appropriate level of detailed knowledge about a single community may require as much or more information as a typical collection of national aggregate statistics.

DISAGGREGATION OF SPECIAL POPULATIONS

Disaggregations of population data generally employ a few conventional variables: age, gender, race and ethnicity, socioeconomic status, education, and location (urban, suburban, rural).

Age

Clearly, youth is the category of age wherein prevention of initial drug use is most relevant, as discussed above. Although experimentation starts in early adolescence and prevalence of current use peaks in the mid-twenties, most of the abuse and dependence is found in older groups—DAWN data shows that the peak ages for emergency room episodes are 20-29 (38.4 percent of all episodes in 1988) and 30-39 (32.2. percent) (Adams et al., 1990). These figures vary somewhat by drug: cocaine cases are highest among the age 20-29 group (48.1 percent), next highest in the age 30-39 group (35.8 percent), and lowest among younger people (6.9 percent). Heroin cases are highest in the age 30-39 group (50.5 percent), next highest in the age 20-29 group (28.8 percent), and lowest among younger people (less than 2 percent). Thus, the profile for heroin indicates a somewhat older population involved with abuse and dependence, compared with cocaine. Regarding alcohol and tobacco, which are initiated at young ages, alcohol requires many years of heavy drinking for the most serious physical consequences to occur (there being two very significant exceptions: traumatic injuries resulting from vehicle crashes and interpersonal violence, both of which are promoted by undercontrolled heavy drinking); and the most devastating consequences from tobacco use generally occur only after many years of use.

Race and Ethnicity

A serious paradox is found in data relating race and ethnicity to drug behavior. National-level population surveys generally show small differences in rates of drug taking among major racial and ethnic groups (e.g., white, Hispanic, black). Both of NIDA's major surveys indicate that cumulative drug taking is lower among young black respondents than among young white respondents, as shown in Table 1.4.

In contrast, case indicators such as DAWN, CODAP, criminal justice data, and mortality, morbidity, and treatment data all show substantial overrepresentation of blacks. Public perceptions are further confounded by media coverage that often focuses on associations between drugs and violence among a small segment of young, economically disadvantaged, cocaine-involved Hispanic and black men in large central cities. Since the survey data indicate that the vast majority of young black men neither use nor sell illicit drugs, these findings suggest a phenomenon of two worlds: by and large, blacks are less likely than whites to be involved with drugs, but those who do get involved are far more likely to become dysfunctional. In other words, there are extremes of abstinence and abuse/dependence in the black population (Herd, 1989).

Drug abuse in urban black communities has become a serious problem (Watts and Wright, 1983). A combination of unfavorable factors such as inadequate housing, economic instability, and high crime rates predispose black youth who do use drugs to abuse. Exposure to these broader environmental influences challenges the black community in the process of child and adolescent development (Thompson and Simmons-Cooper, 1988). Similar phenomena may be operating for Hispanics. National household population survey data suggest that Hispanic drug use prevalence is lower than that of whites overall—except for slightly higher levels of cocaine—but Hispanics are overrepresented in drug treatment and criminal justice statistics (e.g., Hubbard et al., 1989; Adams et al., 1990).

However, as with overall general population figures, these global characterizations mask important variations within groups. Gender differences, for example, tend to be larger within Hispanic groups than for whites and Native Americans; for blacks they are intermediate between the two (NIDA, 1991a). Hispanic groups in particular display very different patterns depending on their specific originating culture; for example, Cubans in the

TABLE 1.4   Lifetime and Past Year Use of Any Illicit Drug[a], by Race
and Age, National Household Survey of Drug Abuse, 1990

Age	White	Hispanic	Black
Lifetime Use			
12-17	24.0	21.1	20.5
18-25	59.3	47.3	47.6
26-34	67.6	45.0	53.7
35+	26.0	22.8	28.9
Past Year Use			
12-17	16.9	17.0	12.7
18-25	30.2	27.3	24.4
26-34	22.4	20.1	24.0
35+	5.7	5.5	8.3

[a]Marijuana, cocaine, heroin, hallucinogens, inhalants, nonmedical use of psychotherapeutics.

SOURCE: National Institute on Drug Abuse (1991a).

United States have generally lower drug use rates than Mexican or other
Latin Americans (Austin and Gilbert, 1989; Bachman et al., 1991; Wallace
and Bachman, 1991; Barnes and Welte, 1987; Newcomb et al., 1987; Oetting
and Beauvis, 1990).

The issue of ethnic variations in drug use is related to a point made
above: that national statistics may not reflect the situation in any particular
community. Because of major demographic changes in recent years, some
geographical regions have especially high densities of specific ethnic populations. For example, in 1990 Hispanics constituted approximately 9 percent of the U.S. population, and 16 percent of this group was located in Los
Angeles. Two-thirds of the Cuban population lives in Miami. A substantial
majority of mainland Puerto Ricans live in New York State and New Jersey.
Many, although not all, Native Americans are geographically removed from
the mainstream population by virtue of the fact that they live on reservations. These geographical and cultural groupings have important implications for prevention efforts and, indeed, for understanding and interpreting
epidemiological data.

Socioeconomic and Economic Factors

Among adolescents and younger adults, impairment is highest among
the least advantaged portions of the population (Simcha-Fagan et al., 1986).
One important segment of society is represented by those who fail to complete high school (Holmberg, 1985; Mensch and Kandel, 1988). This seg-

ment is perennially underemployed and overrepresented in all the indicators of public health and criminal justice problems (Clayton and Tuchfield, 1982; McBride and McCoy, 1982). Over 40 percent of prison inmates in a California prison reported use of cocaine or heroin in the 3 years preceding incarceration (Peterson and Braiker, 1980). Similarly, 83 percent of violent offenders were using drugs daily in the month prior to their committing the offense (Chaiken and Chaiken, 1982). The significance of social environmental factors is given substantial attention in Chapter 2.

However, one of the problems for researchers who attempt to understand drug abuse across and within social classes is that social and economic divisions within the population are not easily understood. The most commonly used measure of social economic status (SES) and the indices derived from SES, such as Duncan's Social Economic Index (SEI) (Hauser and Featherman, 1977) and Hollingshead's (1957) class divisions, were initially developed in the 1950s on the basis of community studies dating back to the 1920s. Ethnographic studies were done in the first half of this century to generate insight about community. They consistently showed that differences in income, occupational status, and education were not the only ways that people drew social lines and perceived themselves and others. These three variables were only the easiest to quantify and compare. Urban communities today are more complex and diverse than they were in the 1920s or 1950s (Green and Simons-Morton, 1991). Yet SES is still used in drug abuse research as the major measure of social boundaries and basis for comparison. It is not an invalid basis, but it sweeps together many culturally specific differences that are very important.

Studies of the clinical and environmental etiology of drug abuse within specific communities and specific segments of the population require insight about social and economic divisions as well as how communities organize themselves and perceive their differences. These kinds of insights cannot be realized or measured by SES alone. Clearly, survey research and sophisticated statistical analysis are limited when the subject population is covert. It is difficult to take representative random samples of fugitive populations, and not enough is known about them to ask all the right questions. Limited access and limited insight restrict the quality and scope of quantitative approaches and call for qualitative research methods, such as ethnography, to contribute in their own right and as a basis for improving quantitative work.

SUMMARY

Research on the nature of the drug problem in America presents a picture of "two worlds." In one, measured by survey data on individuals in school classrooms and households, illicit drug use is not confined to or even particularly prominent in any one social class, economic stratum, race, or ethnic group, although any experience with drugs is self-reported more frequently by the wealthy than the less wealthy and more by whites than Hispanics or blacks. In this world, the drug problem has a remarkably uniform appearance: the sequence of introduction to different drugs seems universal; the diagnostic categories of use, abuse, and dependence are recurrently serviceable; and with regard to the grossest patterns—any use of illicit drugs versus abstinence—the major subgroups of society, in terms of race, ethnicity, and social class, are rather consistent. This world of low-intensity consumption shows steady and cumulatively very marked declines in the prevalence of marijuana use since the late 1970s and of cocaine since the middle 1980s; heroin use is so rare as to be barely measurable.

The other world is that of emergency rooms, morgues, drug clinics, juvenile detention centers, jails, and prisons, in which indicators of intensive drug consumption (abuse and dependence) are collected. When we look closely at the more extreme drug patterns of abuse and dependence, we see a variety of behaviors and consequences that separate into very different levels and follow very distinct trends in different subpopulations compared with each other and with the general population. The poor predominate, blacks and Hispanics appearing in numbers much higher than their household or school proportions; marijuana and heroin use are common (though less so in some areas than in the 1970s); and cocaine use increased explosively throughout the 1980s and simply leveled off at high levels in the 1990s.

Reconciling these two worlds is a major challenge for research. It may be that the processes involved in use, abuse, and dependence (that is, the probabilistic relations of one stage to another and one drug to other drugs) may differ from one population group to another. We need longitudinal studies that are selected so as to be rich in high-risk youth so that we can gain a much better understanding of group as well as individual differences in pathways to and away from drug problems. Researchers need to coordinate their work so that information collected in the two worlds—in households and schools versus hospitals and jails—provides some common points of reference on key items, for example, current probation or parole status and number of hospital visits in the past 12 months. And federal agencies need to place much higher priority on making important national data bases, such as DAWN, DUF, and the household and senior surveys, accessible to a broad range of researchers so they can be used to advance knowledge as well as to keep annual scorecards on a few key indicators.

Moreover, dependence and abuse tend to cluster with many other behaviors that are defined as serious problems. According to Jessor (1983), drug use represents part of a syndrome of problem behavior. Youth who use drugs are more likely to be involved in delinquency and precocious sexual activity (Jessor and Jessor, 1977). The relationship between adolescent drug abuse and delinquency is well established; frequent use and abuse of drugs are more common among youth involved in chronic delinquent activities than other adolescents (see Hawkins, Lishner, Jensen and Catalano, 1987). In the National Youth Study, one-half of serious juvenile offenders were also multiple illicit drug users (Elliott and Huizinga, 1984). Research findings indicate that drug use and criminal behavior represent manifestations of social involvement in the drug-using subculture (Faupel, 1988). In fact, subpopulations involved most heavily in drug consumption tend to be afflicted with a whole variety of health and behavioral dysfunctions, so the drug diagnosis may or may not be primary or defining. The most visibly damaging drug behavior and the violence associated with it occur among the economically disadvantaged.

Different kinds of prevention opportunities arise in relation to how individuals behave across time, how the behaviors and consequences are distributed across social groups, and how they cluster with other problems. These results suggest that there needs to be more examination of specific factors, both individual and environmental, that affect onset, progression, and problem clustering, and then to develop lessons of this knowledge for intervention planning and research.

REFERENCES

Adams, E.
   1990   Interview. *DAWN Briefings* 6(4):5.
Adams, E.H., A.J. Blanken, L.D. Ferguson, and A. Kopstein
   1990   *Overview of Selected Drug Trends.* Rockville, Md.: National Institute on Drug Abuse.
Akers, R.L., M.D. Krohn, L. Lanza-Kaduco, and M. Radosevich
   1979   Social learning and deviant behavior: a specific test of a general theory. *American Sociological Review* 44(4):636-755.
American Psychiatric Association
   1987   *Diagnostic and Statistical Manual of Mental Disorders*, 3rd ed., revised. Washington, D.C.: American Psychiatric Association.
Aquilino, W.S., and L.A. Losciuto
   1990   Effects of interview mode on self-reported drug use. *Public Opinion Quarterly* 56:362-295.
Austin, G.A., and M.J. Gilbert
   1989   Substance abuse among Latino youth. *Prevention Research Update* 3:1-26.
Bachman, J.G., J.M. Wallace, Jr., P.M. O'Malley, L.D. Johnston, C.L. Kurth, and H.W. Neighbors
   1991   Racial/ethnic differences in smoking, drinking, and illicit drug use among American high school seniors, 1976-89. *American Journal of Public Health* 81:372-377.
Barnes, G.M., and J.M. Welte
   1987   Patterns and predictors of alcohol use among 7-12th grade students in New York State. *Journal of Studies on Alcohol* 47:53-62.

Barth, R.P.
1991   Educational implications of prenatally drug-exposed children. *Social Work in Education* 13(2):130-136.

Blanken, A.
1989   Epidemiologic Trends in Drug Abuse. In *Proceedings of the Community Epidemiology Work Group: June 1989.* Rockville, Md.: National Institute on Drug Abuse.

Block, R.K., S. Farnham, K. Braverman, R. Noyes, Jr., and M.M. Ghoneim
1990   Long-term marijuana use and subsequence effects on learning and cognitive functions related to school achievement: preliminary study. Pp. 96-111 in J.W. Spencer and J.J. Boren, eds., *Residual Effects of Abused Drugs on Behavior.* NIDA Research Monograph 101. Rockville, Md.: National Institute on Drug Abuse.

Booth, R., S. Koester, J.T. Brewster, W.W. Weibel, and R.B. Fritz
1991   Intravenous drug users and AIDS: risk behaviors. *American Journal of Drug and Alcohol Abuse* 17(3):337-353.

Buchanan, D.
1991   How teens think about drugs: insights from moral reasoning and social bonding theory. *International Quarterly of Community Health Education* 11:315-332.

Buchanan, D.R.
1992   An uneasy alliance: combining qualitative and quantitative research methods. *Health Education Quarterly* 19:117-135.

Centers for Disease Control
1987   HIV infection prevalence among groups at recognized risk. *Morbidity and Mortality Weekly Report* 36(Suppl. S-6). Atlanta, Ga.: Centers for Disease Control.

Centers for Disease Control
1990   *HIV/AIDS Surveillance.* April. Table 4. Atlanta, Ga.: Centers for Disease Control.

Chaiken, J., and M.R. Chaiken
1982   *Varieties of Criminal Behavior.* Santa Monica, Calif.: The Rand Corporation.

Chasnoff, I.J., ed.
1989   *Drugs, Alcohol, Pregnancy and Parenting.* Hingham, Mass.: Kluwer Academic Publishers.

Chasnoff, I.J., D.R. Griffith, S. MacGregor, K. Dirkes, and K.A. Burns
1989   Temporal patterns of cocaine use in pregnancy. *Journal of the American Medical Association* 261(12):1741-1744.

Chasnoff, I.J., H.J. Landress, and M.E. Barrett
1990   The prevalence of illicit-drug or alcohol use during pregnancy and discrepancies in mandatory reporting in Pinellas County, Florida. *New England Journal of Medicine* 322:1202-1206.

Chavez, G.F., J. Mulinare, and J.F. Cordero
1989   Maternal cocaine use during early pregnancy as a risk factor for congenital urogenital anomalies. *Journal of the American Medical Association* 262(6):795-798.

Chitwood, D.D., C.B. McCoy, and M. Comerford
1990   Risk behavior of intravenous drug users. Pp. 120-133 in C.G. Leukefeld et al., eds., *AIDS and Intravenous Drug Use.* New York: Hemisphere Publishing Corporation.

Clayton, R.R., and H.L. Voss
1981   *Young Men and Drugs in Manhattan: A Causal Analysis.* NIDA Research Monograph 19. Rockville, Md.: National Institute on Drug Abuse.

Clayton, R.R., and B.S. Tuchfield
1982   The drug-crime debate: obstacles to understanding the relationship. *Journal of Drug Issues* 12(2):153-166.

Clayton, R.R., H.L. Voss, and L.A. LoSciuto
  1987   Gateway drugs: what are the stages people go through in becoming drug abusers. *Pharmacy Times* 53(March):38-35.
Community Epidemiology Working Group
  1992a   *Epidemiologic Trends in Drug Abuse: Proceedings, Community Epidemiology Work Group, December, 1991.* DHHS Pub. No. (ADM)92-1918. Rockville, Md.: National Institute on Drug Abuse.
Community Epidemiology Working Group
  1992b   *Epidemiologic Trends in Drug Abuse: Proceedings, Community Epidemiology Work Group, June, 1992.* DHHS Pub. No. (ADM)92-1958. Rockville, Md.: National Institute on Drug Abuse.
Courtwright, D.T.
  1992   A century of American narcotic policy. Pp. 1-62 in D.R. Gerstein and H.J. Harwood, eds., *Treating Drug Problems*, Vol. 2. Committee for the Substance Abuse Coverage Study, Institute of Medicine. Washington, D.C.: National Academy Press.
Crider, R.A.
  1985   Heroin incidence: a trend comparison between national household survey data and indicator data. Pp. 125-140 in B.A. Rouse et al., eds., *Self-Report Methods of Estimating Drug Use: Meeting Current Challenges to Validity.* NIDA Research Monograph 57. Rockville, Md.: National Institute on Drug Abuse.
Dembo, R., L. Willrams, J. Schmeidler, E.D. Wish, A. Getreu, and E. Berry
  1991   Juvenile crime and drug abuse: a prospective study of high risk youth. *Journal of Addictive Diseases* 11:5-31.
Donovan, J.E., and R. Jessor
  1985   Structure of problem behavior in adolescence and young adulthood. *Journal of Consulting and Clinical Psychology* 53:890-904.
Duncan, D.F.
  1988   *Epidemiology: Basis for Disease Prevention and Health Promotion.* New York: Macmillan Publishing Co.
Duster, T.
  1970   *The Legislation of Morality.* New York: Free Press.
Elliott, D.S., and D. Huizinga
  1984   The Relationship Between Delinquent Behavior and ADM Problem Behaviors. Paper prepared for the ADAMHA/OJJDP State of the Art Research Conference on Juvenile Offenders with Serious Drug/Alcohol and Mental Health Problems, Bethesda, Md.
Faupel, C.E.
  1988   Heroin use, crime and employment status. *Journal of Drug Issues* 18(3):467-479.
Feldman, H.W.
  1968   Ideological supports to becoming and remaining a heroin addict. *Journal of Health and Social Behavior* 9:121-139.
Feucht, T.E., R.C. Stephens, and S.W. Roman
  1990   The sexual behavior of intravenous drug users: assessing the risk of sexual transmission of HIV. *Journal of Drug Issues* 20(2):195-213.
Forman, S.G., and J.A. Linney
  1991   Increasing the validity of self-report data in effectiveness trials. In C.G. Leukefeld and W.J. Bukoski, eds., *Drug Abuse Prevention Intervention Research: Methodologic Issues.* NIDA Research Monograph 107. Rockville, Md.: National Institute on Drug Abuse.
Frank, B.
  1985   Telephone surveying for drug abuse: methodological issues and an application.

In B.A. Rouse et al., eds., *Self-Report Methods of Estimating Drug Use: Meeting Current Challenges to Validity*. NIDA Research Monograph 57. Rockville, Md.: National Institute on Drug Abuse.

Friedman, G.H., and R.S. Klein
1987   Transmission of the human immunodeficiency virus. *New England Journal of Medicine* 317:1125-1135.

Fullilove, M.T., and R.E. Fullilove
1989   Intersecting epidemics: black teen crack use and sexually transmitted disease. *Journal of the American Medicine Women's Association* 44:146-153.

Gerstein, D.R., and H.J. Harwood, eds.
1990   *Treating Drug Problems*, Vol. 1. Committee for the Substance Abuse Coverage Study, Institute of Medicine. Washington, D.C.: National Academy Press.

Green, L.W., and D. Simons-Morton
1991   Education and lifestyle determinants of health and disease. Pp. 181-196 in W.W. Holland, R. Detels, and G. Knox, eds., *Oxford Textbook of Public Health: Influences of Public Health*, 2nd ed., Vol. 1. New York: Oxford University Press.

Hamburg, B.A., H.C. Kraemer, and W. Jahnke
1975   A hierarchy of drug use in adolescence: behavioral and attitudinal correlates of substantial drug use. *American Journal of Psychiatry* 132(11):1155-1163.

Harwood, H., D.M. Napolitano, P.L. Christensen, and J.J. Collins
1984   Economic Costs to Society of Alcohol and Drug Abuse and Mental Illness: 1980. Report to the Alcohol, Drug Abuse and Mental Health Administration. Research Triangle Institute, Research Triangle Park, N.C.

Hauser, R., and D. Featherman
1977   *The Process of Stratification: Trends and Analysis*. New York: Academic Press.

Hawkins, J.D., D.M. Lishner, J.M. Jensen, and R.F. Catalano
1987   Delinquents and drugs: what the evidence suggests about treatment programming. Pp. 81-131 in B.S. Brown and A.R. Mills, eds., *Youth at High Risk for Substance Abuse*. Rockville, Md.: National Institute on Drug Abuse.

Henningfield, J.E.
1984   Behavioral pharmacology of cigarette smoking. Pp. 131-210 in T. Thompson et al., eds., *Advances in Behavioral Pharmacology*, Vol. 4. Hillsdale, N.J.: Lawrence Erlbaum Associates.

Henningfield, J.E., R.R. Clayton, and W. Pollin
1990   The involvement of tobacco in alcoholism and illicit drug use. *British Journal of Addiction* 85:279-292.

Herd, D.
1989   The epidemiology of drinking patterns and alcohol related problems among U.S. Blacks. Pp. 3-50 in D.L. Spiegler et al., eds., *Alcohol Use Among U.S. Ethnic Minorities*. NIAAA DHHS Pub. No. (ADM)89-1435. Washington, D.C.: U.S. Government Printing Office.

Hoegsberg, B., T. Dotson, O. Abulafia et al.
1989   Social, Sexual and Drug Use Profile of HIV(+) and HIV(-) Women with PID. Paper presented at the V International Conference on AIDS, Montreal.

Hollingshead, A.B.
1957   *The Two-Factor Index of Social Position*. New Haven, Conn.: privately published.

Holmberg, M.B.
1985   Longitudinal studies of drug abuse in a fifteen-year-old population. *Acta Psychiatrica Scandinavica* 16:129-136.

Hubbard, R.L., M.E. Marsden, J.V. Rachal, H.J. Harwood, E.R. Cavanaugh, and H.M. Ginzburg
1989   *Drug Abuse Treatment: A National Study of Effectiveness*. Chapel Hill: The University of North Carolina Press.

Institute of Medicine
1989   *Prevention and Treatment of Alcohol Problems: Research Opportunities.* Washington, D.C.: National Academy Press.

Jaffe, J.H.
1990   Drug addiction and drug abuse. Pp. 522-573 in *Goodman and Gilman's the Pharmacological Basis of Therapeutics*, 8th ed. New York: Pergamon Press.

Jessor, R.
1983   A psychosocial perspective on adolescent substance use. In I.F. Litt, ed., *Adolescent Substance Abuse: Report on the Fourteenth Ross Roundtable.* Columbus, Ohio: Ross Laboratories.

Jessor, R.
1991   Risk behavior in adolescence: a psychosocial framework for understanding and action. *Journal of Adolescent Health Care* 12:597-605.

Jessor, R., and S.L. Jessor
1977   *Problem Behavior and Psychosocial Development: A Longitudinal Study of Youth.* New York: Academic Press.

Johnston, L.D., and P.M. O'Malley
1986   Why do the nation's students use drugs and alcohol? Self-reported reasons from nine national surveys. *Journal of Drug Issues* 16(1):29-66.

Johnston, L.D., P.M. O'Malley, and J.G. Bachman
1991a   *Drug Use, Drinking, and Smoking: National Survey Results from High School, College, and Young Adult Populations: 1975-1990. Vol. 1. High School Seniors.* DHHS Pub. No. (ADM) 91-1813. Rockville, Md.: National Institute on Drug Abuse.

Johnston, L.D., P.M. O'Malley, and J.G. Bachman
1991b   *Drug Use, Drinking, and Smoking: National Survey Results from High School, College, and Young Adult Populations: 1975-1990, Vol. 2. College Students and Young Adults.* DHHS Pub. No. (ADM) 91-1835. Rockville, Md.: National Institute on Drug Abuse.

Jonsen, A., ed.
1993   *The Social Impact of AIDS.* Panel on Monitoring the Social Impact of AIDS, Committee on AIDS Research and the Behavior, Social and Statistical Sciences, National Research Council. Washington, D.C.: National Academy Press.

Kandel, D.B.
1975   Stages of adolescent involvement in drug use. *Science* 190:912-914.

Kandel, D.B., and J.A. Logan
1984   Patterns of drug use from adolescence to young adulthood: I. Periods of risk for initiation, continuation, and discontinuation. *American Journal of Public Health* 74(7):660-665.

Kandel, D.B., E. Single, and R.C. Kessler
1976   The epidemiology of drug use among New York state high school students: distribution, trends, and change in rates of use. *American Journal of Public Health* 66:43-53.

Kandel, D.B., M. Davies, M. Karus, and K. Yamaguchi
1986   The consequences in young adulthood of adolescent drug involvement: an overview. *Archives of General Psychiatry* 43(8):746-754.

Koren, G., K. Graham, H. Shear, and T. Einarson
1989   Bias against the null hypothesis: the reproductive hazards of cocaine. *Lancet* 16:1440-1442.

Kusserow, R.P.
1990   *Cocaine Exposed Infants.* Office of Inspector General. Washington, D.C.: U.S. Department of Health and Human Services.

Last, J.M., and R.B. Wallace
1991   *Maxcy-Rosenau Public Health and Preventive Medicine*, 13th ed. Norwalk, Calif.: Appleton-Century-Crofts.

LeBlanc, P.E., A.J. Parekh, B. Naso, et al.
1987   Effects of intrauterine exposure to alkaloidal cocaine (crack). *American Journal of Disease in Childhood* 141:937-938.

Levison, P.K., D.R. Gerstein, and D.R. Maloff
1983   *Commonalities in Substance Abuse and Habitual Behavior*. Committee of Substance Abuse and Habitual Behavior, National Research Council. Lexington, Mass.: Lexington Books.

Lidz, C., and A. Walker
1980   *Heroin, Deviants and Morality*. Beverly Hills, Calif.: Sage Publications.

McAuliffe, W.E., P. Breer, N.W. Ahmadifer, and C. Spino
1991   Assessment of drug abuser treatment needs in Rhode Island. *American Journal of Public Health* 81:365-370.

McBride, D.C., and C.B. McCoy
1982   Crime and drugs: the issues and literature. *Journal of Drug Issues* 12(2):137-151.

McKirnan, D.J., and T. Johnston
1986   Alcohol and drug use among "street" adolescents. *Addictive Behaviors* 11:201-205.

Mensch, B.S., and D.B. Kandel
1988   Do job conditions influence the use of drugs? *Journal of Health and Social Behavior* 29(June):169-184.

Miller, J.D.
1985   The nominative technique: a new method of estimating prevalence. In B.A. Rouse, N.J. Kozel, and L.G. Richards, eds., *Self-Report Methods of Estimating Drug Use: Meeting Current Challenges to Validity*. NIDA Research Monograph 57. Rockville, Md.: National Institute on Drug Abuse.

Moncher, M.S., G.W. Holden, and S.P. Schinke
1991   Psychosocial correlates of adolescent substance use: a review of current etiological constructs. *International Journal of the Addictions* 26(4):377-414.

Murray, D., and C.L. Perry
1984   Functional Meaning of Adolescent Drug Use. Paper presented at a meeting of the American Psychological Association, Toronto.

Murray, D.M., and C.L. Perry
1987   The measurement of substance use among adolescents: when is the "bogus pipeline" method needed? *Addictive Behaviors* 12(3):225-233.

Musto, D.
1987   *The American Disease*, 2nd ed. New Haven, Conn.: Yale University Press.

Nathan, P.E.
1990   Residual effects of alcohol. Pp. 112-123 in J.W. Spencer and J.J. Boren, eds., *Residual Effects of Abused Drugs on Behavior*. NIDA Research Monograph 101. Rockville, Md.: National Institute on Drug Abuse.

National Institute on Drug Abuse
1991a   *National Household Survey on Drug Abuse: Populations Estimates 1990*. DHHS Pub. No. (ADM)91-1732. Rockville, Md.: National Institute on Drug Abuse.

National Institute on Drug Abuse
1991b   *National Household Survey on Drug Abuse: Main Findings 1990*. DHHS Pub. No. (ADM) 91-1778. Rockville, Md.: National Institute on Drug Abuse.

Newcomb, M.D., and P.M. Bentler
1986   Frequency and sequence of drug use: a longitudinal study from early adolescence to young adulthood. *Journal of Drug Education* 16(2):101-120.

Newcomb, M.D., E. Maddahain, R. Skager, and P.M. Bentler
  1987 Substance abuse and psychosocial risk factors among teenagers: association with sex, age, ethnicity, and type of school. *American Journal of Drug and Alcohol Abuse* 13:413-433.
New York Times
  1990 Washington Talk: Drug War Underlines Fickleness of Public. Sept. 6:PA22.
O'Donnell, J.A., and R.R. Clayton
  1982 The stepping stone hypothesis—marijuana, heroin, and causality. *Chemical Dependencies: Behavioral and Biomedical Issues* 4:229-241.
O'Donnell, J.A., H.L. Voss, R.R. Clayton, G.T. Slatin, and R. Room
  1976 *Young Men and Drugs: A Nationwide Survey.* NIDA Research Monograph 5. Rockville, Md.: National Institute on Drug Abuse.
Oetting, E.R., and F. Beauvis
  1990 Adolescent drug use: findings of national and local surveys. *Journal of Consulting and Clinical Psychology* 58(4):385-394.
O'Neil, J.A., and C. Visher
  1992 *Drug Use Forecasting Quarterly Report,* 2nd Quarter, 1991. Washington, D.C.: U.S. Department of Justice.
Pederson, L.L., and N.M. Lefcoe
  1985 Cross-sectional analysis of variables related to cigarette smoking in late adolescence. *Journal of Drug Education* 15(3):225-240.
Peterson, L., and H.B. Braiker
  1980 *Doing Crime: A Survey of California Prison Inmates.* Santa Monica, Calif.: The Rand Corporation.
President's Advisory Commission on Narcotics and Drug Abuse
  1963 *Final Report.* Washington, D.C.: U.S. Government Printing Office.
Puccio, P.S., and R.S. Simeone
  1991 *Drug and Other Substance Use Among School Children in New York State.* Albany, N.Y.: New York State Division of Substance Abuse Services.
Rice, D.P., S. Kelman, L. Miller, and S. Dunmeyer
  1990 The Economic Costs of Alcohol, Drug Abuse, and Mental Illness—1985. Institute for Health and Aging, University of California, San Francisco.
Rogers, E.M.
  1983 *Diffusion of Innovations,* 3rd ed. New York: Free Press.
Rouse, B.A., N.J. Coxal, and L.G. Richards, eds.
  1985 *Self-Report Methods of Estimating Drug Use: Meeting Current Challenges to Validity.* NIDA Research Monograph 57. Rockville, Md.: National Institute on Drug Abuse.
Siegel, R.K.
  1992 Repeating cycles of cocaine use and abuse. Pp. 289-316 in D.R. Gerstein and H.J. Harwood, eds., *Treating Drug Problems,* Vol. II. Committee for the Substance Abuse Coverage Study, National Research Council. Washington, D.C.: National Academy Press.
Simcha-Fagen, O., J.C. Gersten, and T.S. Langer
  1986 Early precursors and concurrent correlates of patterns of illicit drug use in adolescence. *Journal of Drug Issues* 16(1):7-28.
Simons-Morton, B.G., S.G. Brink, D.G. Simons-Morton, R. McIntyre, M. Chapman, J. Longoria, and G.S. Parcel
  1989 An ecological approach to the prevention of injuries due to drinking and driving. *Health Education Quarterly* 16:397-411.
Sirken, M.L.
  1975 Network surveys of rare and sensitive conditions. Pp. 31-32 in *Advances in Health*

Survey Research Methods. Proceedings. Hyattsville, Md.: National Center on Health Statistics.

Spencer, B.D.
1989   On the accuracy of current estimates of the numbers of intravenous drug users. Pp. 429-446 in C.F. Turner et al., eds., *AIDS: Sexual Behavior and Intravenous Drug Use.* Committee on AIDS Research and the Behavioral, Social and Statistical Sciences. Washington, D.C.: National Academy Press.

Spencer, J.W., and J.J. Boren, eds.
1990   *Residual Effects of Abused Drugs on Behavior.* NIDA Research Monograph 101. Rockville, Md.: National Institute on Drug Abuse.

Thompson, T., and C. Simmons-Cooper
1988   Chemical dependency treatment and black adolescents. *Journal of Drug Issues* 18(1):21-31.

Turner, C.F., H.G. Miller, and L.E. Moses
1989   *AIDS: Sexual Behavior and Intravenous Drug Use.* Committee on AIDS Research and the Behavioral, Social, and Statistical Sciences, Commission on Behavioral and Social Sciences and Education, National Research Council. Washington, D.C.: National Academy Press.

Wallace, J.M., Jr., and J.G. Bachman
1991   Explaining racial/ethnic differences in adolescent drug use: the impact of background and lifestyle. *Social Problems* 38(3):333-357.

Warner, S.L.
1965   Randomized response: a survey technique for estimating evasive answer bias. *Journal of the American Statistical Association* 60:63-69.

Watts, T.D., and W. Wright, Jr.
1983   *Black Alcoholism: Toward a Comprehensive Understanding.* Springfield, Ill.: Charles C Thomas Publishing.

Werch, C.E., D.R. Gorman, P.J. Marty, J. Forbess, and B. Brown
1987   Effects of the bogus pipeline on enhancing validity of self-reported adolescent drug use measures. *Journal of School Health* 57:232-236.

White House
1992   *National Drug Control Strategy: A Nation Responds to Drug Use—Budget Summary.* Washington, D.C.: White House.

World Health Organization
1992   *International Statistical Classification of Diseases, Injuries, and Causes of Death,* 10th ed. Geneva: World Health Organization.

Yamaguchi, K., and D.B. Kandel
1984a   Patterns of drug use from adolescence to young adulthood: II. Sequences of progression. *American Journal of Public Health* 74(7):668-672.

Yamaguchi, K., and D.B. Kandel
1984b   Patterns of drug use from adolescence to young adulthood: III. Predictors of progression. *American Journal of Public Health* 74(7):673-681.

Zuckerman, B., D.A. Frank, R. Hingson, and H. Amara
1989   Effects of maternal marijuana and cocaine use on fetal growth. *New England Journal of Medicine* 320(12):762-768.

2

Concepts of Prevention

To prevent drug abuse, the central question is: What individual and group factors need to be considered in designing interventions to be effective? To answer that question, a series of related questions have been investigated: What *elements* affect the probability of onset, progression, severity, and cessation of drug use, abuse, and dependence? By what *mechanisms* do these factors work, in what combinations, and with what degrees of strength or determinacy? What *interventions* can be used to subject these probabilistic factors to preventive change?

INTRODUCTION

The research in this field has had to cope with great complexity, involving multiple causal and conditioning pathways and factors that are influential in some populations or environments but that appear far less salient in others. In trying to untangle this complexity, research has followed a number of paths, some of which were ultimately abandoned as unfruitful. Over time, the field has increasingly become oriented to a few systematic approaches that have survived tests of theoretical coherence and empirical plausibility. Although these approaches are not antagonistic or contradictory, they differ dramatically in emphasis. A more encompassing synthesis or integration of approaches is not realistically in view. Nevertheless, an overarching, three-part conceptual framework is helpful in understanding the current approaches, and it provides a good basis for considering their differences and commonalities. We refer to three general concepts as predisposing, enabling, and reinforcing elements.

Predisposing elements, the first part of the framework, are comprised of internalized individual characteristics (also called diatheses) and environmental exposures (conditions). Predisposing elements are in effect prior to the first encounter or opportunity to try illicit drugs. Predispositional logic holds that some subsets of individuals, by virtue of factors that they have acquired or been exposed to, are more vulnerable or more resistant to drug use, abuse, or dependence than individuals without such factors, or with less of them, all other things being equal. Potential predisposing elements may be genetically transmitted vulnerability in the form of certain temperamental or physiological characteristics; developmental deficits, such as failures in early socialization or a lack of self-esteem, which imply that interaction within the family is an important locus of concern; knowledge and beliefs concerning the hazards of drugs; the individual's own perceptions of a drug's ability to harm; moral beliefs and attitudes about drug consumption; or the individual's social circumstances and prospects irrespective of family interaction.

Second are enabling elements. These are decision-making and economic or other circumstances relating directly to individual behavior in the situation of opportunity to consume a drug. The major enablers are of two kinds: (1) the availability and accessibility of drugs and prevention or treatment resources in the community and (2) the individual's skills to define and respond autonomously and effectively to problem situations such as the ones that drug availability presents.

Knowledge or belief structures, self-perceptions, and skills may be transmitted interpersonally or through mass media. The distribution of both predisposing and enabling elements tends to be associated with socioeconomic class and ethnicity. The relationship of predisposing and enabling elements may be critical to understanding why the rates of onset of drug use may be similar in different groups but then diverge into sharply different rates of drug abuse and dependence.

Third are reinforcing elements, which are the environmental (especially social and economic) contingencies that attach to drug-related behavior. Reinforcement may result from social recognition by a significant other or members of an important reference group, in the form of giving or withholding approval (praise, prestige, esteem), disapproval (complaint, ridicule, or dislike), or intimacy; or earning money or acquiring property as a result of drug-related income. Major significant others and groups include parents (whose influence declines over time), peers (whose influence increases from childhood to adolescence); teachers; and job supervisors and coworkers (including military peers and superiors). Parents may retain greater influence than peers in some families. Like enabling elements, social reinforcers are distributed differently in different socioeconomic classes, ethnic groups, and residential zones (Green and Kreuter, 1991; Gottlieb and Green, 1987; Heckler, 1985; Jacob, 1987; Thomas, 1990).

There are four major conceptual approaches to prevention: risk-factor, developmental, social influence, and community-specific. We briefly define each of these approaches in the next few pages. We then proceed in the balance of the chapter to present a more thorough review of the respective literatures of the first three approaches. Since the community-specific approach is still largely outside the drug prevention research literature, we defer discussion of this approach to the appendix.

The Risk Factor Approach

Three major schools of thinking and associated research about prevention emphasize one or more of these concepts of predisposing, enabling, and reinforcing elements. The first school speaks principally in terms of *risk factors*, a concept that is used extensively in the epidemiology of cardiovascular, cancer, and other chronic diseases (Bry et al., 1982; Newcomb et al., 1987). This is the most comprehensive approach in terms of the range and number of factors considered; it is also the least theoretically structured and the least empirically focused.

A risk factor is any observable (measurable) characteristic of the individual (including duration of exposure to specified environmental conditions) that has been shown to correlate significantly (in population or case-control studies) with a criterion behavior or outcome—in this case, with the onset of illicit drug use, some threshold level of consumption, or the clinical occurrence of drug abuse or dependence. This specification makes the risk factor model more empirical than theoretical. The risk factor must precede or at least occur simultaneously with the drug behavior; that is, a risk factor must be a potential cause or precursor, not a direct or indirect effect or symptom, of the criterion behavior. Reciprocal causation between risk factors and criterion behaviors is not precluded; in fact, as discussed below, a mutually reinforcing feedback among problem behaviors is the common pattern. For example, the desire for peer approval may predispose a teenager to try marijuana with her friends, the reduced inhibition and the relaxation felt during use reinforces the behavior and predisposes her to another opportunity to use. Most of the risk factors studied, in terms of the conceptual framework just reviewed, count as predisposing elements.

Interventions to prevent drug use following the risk factor approach tend to emphasize educational approaches to modify self-esteem, specific beliefs and attitudes concerning drug use, and related predisposing factors (Bry et al., 1982; Newcomb et al., 1987). Risk factors are statistical or probabilistic: if an individual "has" the factor, his or her odds (that is, statistical risk) of having the outcome are higher than if the individual does not have the factor, all other things being equal. For example, if John thinks marijuana is harmless, then the odds that he will try it are higher than if he thinks marijuana can hurt him. Risk factors are usually additive: that is, risks add up; the more of them that apply, the more probable it is that the criterion outcome "at risk" will be observed. Some risk factors are easier to change than others, and some risk factors may weigh more heavily (higher zero-order or partial correlations with the criterion) than others. Those that meet both of these criteria become more strategic targets for intervention.

Some risks may interact or have "synergistic" effects, in which one factor statistically multiplies rather than simply adds to the effect of other factors; in other words, a may be a nonsignificant risk factor, b may be a nonsignificant risk factor, but a and b together may be a formidably significant risk factor. Thus, although a may be a significant risk factor, in the absence of b, its effect on drug use is minimal. An open question is whether risk factors are generic (i.e., to many drugs) or specific (to each drug family).

The Developmental Approach

The second school of thought about prevention is based on *developmental theory*. This approach particularly emphasizes the character and dynamics of interaction over time within the family during early childhood and within environments such as the school, especially grades 1-6. It shares with some risk factor theories a concern with early developmental deficits or predisposing factors. It differs, however, from risk factor theories in its heavy concentration on characteristics of the family and school environment that directly reinforce undesirable patterns of affect, belief, or (most important) behavior. Conversely, it also concentrates on environmental reinforcement of the development of positive motivation, educational potential, and prosocial behavior. The developmental approach articulates a more elaborately linked and structured set of factors than risk factor approach. It has a more diffuse target, however; instead of trying to identify and focus on individuals who are "high risk" as the object of preemptive intervention, the developmental approach tends to bracket more inclusive populations and more dimensions of lifestyle or behavior (more than drug use, that is) as the loci of long-term environmental and institutional change.

Social Influence Approaches

The third major school of thought about prevention—really a family of related approaches—involves research on *social influence*. It is the most tightly focused theoretically, and it is population-based. Increasing attention is being given in social influence research to variations among demographic and other groups. It recognizes the important role of peers in the initiation and progression of drug use.

The social influence model is based on four core components: (1) providing information on the negative social and short-term physiological consequences of smoking; (2) providing information on the social influences to smoke—namely, peer, parents, and mass media; (3) correcting inflated perceptions of smoking prevalence; and (4) training, modeling, rehearsal, and reinforcement of methods to resist the social influences to smoke.

Interventions largely concentrate on 6th through 10th grade students and are best known for aiming to prevent the onset of use by modifying enabling factors; in particular, increasing the knowledge of harmful effects and teaching specific *resistance skills* for resisting persuasive messages from peers and mass media. Cigarette smoking is the most thoroughly documented health-related behavior in social influence theory, and most interventions to increase resistance skills were originally developed and tested in the context of preventing the onset of smoking (Evans and Raines, 1982). We have documented the relevance of smoking prevention to illicit drug use prevention in Chapter 1, in the discussion of gateway drugs and the sequence of progression of drug involvement.

An important variation on social influence approaches is the *cognitive-behavioral* model, which is based on the assumption that substance use results from the combined influences of social and psychological factors. Based on work by Schinke and colleagues on pregnancy prevention (Schinke and Gilchrest, 1977; Schinke, 1982), this approach has been adapted to smoking and other substances. The theoretical basis of the model is derived from both developmental and social learning theory. Alcohol and drug use is viewed as instrumental in meeting the developmental needs of youth (e.g., transition marker, reducing stress, peer group acceptance, establishing independence). The strategy for drug prevention emphasizes the development of enabling skills, the acquisition of decision-making and problem-solving skills to equip youth to make informed decisions about alcohol and drug use. The focus is on the development of cognitive, behavioral, and interpersonal skills. The approach is based on five core elements, which:

- deal with a wide range of problem situations through the use of a systematic problem-solving strategy,
- provide accurate information,
- teach coping strategies to relive stress and anxiety,
- develop assertiveness skills, and
- develop self-instructional techniques for behavioral self-control.

A final important stream of work is the life skills approach, which emphasizes the development of general life and coping skills, in addition to skills and knowledge related more directly to resisting peer influences to use substances (Botvin et al., 1980; Botvin and Eng, 1980). The program focuses on teaching cognitive-behavioral skills that remedy psychological or behavioral deficits. The Life Skills Model program consists of three major components. A substance-specific component incorporates most of the information from the social influences approach. A second component addresses developing personal skills such as coping strategies, critical thinking, and decision-making skills and teaches the basic principles of behavior change. A third component develops social skills designed to improve interpersonal functioning.

The Community-Specific Approach

A fourth perspective attempts to encompass all of the prior three. We refer to this as the community-specific prevention approach. Community-specific prevention is receiving major attention in various fields of public health, particularly in preventing cigarette smoking and in controlling risk factors for cardiovascular disease, cancer, AIDS, teenage pregnancy, and other major health or related social problems.

The conceptual foundations of drug abuse prevention historically have been imported from behavioral and social science research on cigarette smoking reduction and public health promotion generally. Large differences in the scale and nature of severe drug problems experienced in different communities makes the community-specific approach seem especially applicable to drug abuse prevention, insofar as it is oriented to investigating population differences and community variations, and to mobilizing resources accordingly. The community-specific approach is, nevertheless, a barely cultivated areas of drug abuse prevention research, within which the published work is not commensurate in scope with the risk-factor, developmental, and social-influence literatures. Therefore, we take this subject up in the appendix, which looks more generally to community-based health education to illuminate this important dimension.

STUDIES OF RISK AND VULNERABILITY

Much research attention has been focused on *risk factors*—variables that exist before or during the typical age of onset of drug use (the second decade of life) and predict an elevated probability of developing abuse or dependence—and on their mirror image, *protective factors*—those that seem to confer a degree of immunity against drug involvement. By and large, risk and protective factors are opposed ends of a set of continua, for example, impulsivity versus planning, strong versus weak family bonding (Jessor et al., 1992). Risk and protective factors thus refer to relative degrees of vulnerability on a set of continua.

Risk and protective factors may be characteristics of the individual or of the environment. Individuals vary greatly in physical and behavioral responses to nearly all health-related exposures or opportunities; they also vary in the environments to which they are exposed. The study of such variations and how they affect the probability of health problems has been immensely important in the history of medicine and public health, so it is no surprise that this approach has been adopted in the drug area (Rennert et al., 1986).

A salient finding about patterns of drug consumption, discussed in the previous chapter, is the fact that a much larger number of individuals use drugs—some very briefly, some intermittently over a longer span of years, some regularly but at a modest level that does not increase over time—than the number who progress to the clinical status of abuse or dependence. The infrequent and/or low-dose use of drugs is not a matter of indifference, because such use is illegal and can have serious consequences. Any level of use generates a degree of risk of progression to abuse or dependence as a result of internal reinforcement, and use by some is likely to model or reinforce abuse and dependence by others. But by definition, the consequences of use are much less hazardous for the individual, on average, than the consequences of abuse and dependence. Although users outnumber drug dependent and abusing individuals, the smaller number of the latter incur the majority of the social costs of drug problems. It is therefore important to give particular attention to the degree to which particular causes increase the probability of abuse or dependence over and above the incidence of drug use per se.

There are indications that the processes leading to use may be differentiated from those leading to abuse and dependence. In particular, unusually early onset of drug use (that is, well before the average age of onset in the population) is a strong correlate of later abuse or dependence, although this is not an infallible marker (Kandel et al., 1986). The early onset of cigarette smoking is of special interest, and early alcohol and marijuana onset are also of concern, because these tend to be gateways to other drugs.

Most studies of drug-related risk factors have been exploratory rather than substantive, that is, they have employed small samples, followed up for abbreviated periods, and have inadequate disaggregation and control for gender, race/ethnicity, and socioeconomic status. There are, however, a few studies large enough to establish with a certain degree of confidence the relative importance of key factors, including longitudinal studies conducted by a number of research teams, including: Judith Brook and colleagues (Brook et al., 1990); Brunswick (1988); Elliott and colleagues (Elliott et al., 1989); Jessor and colleagues (Jessor and Jessor, 1977); Kandel and colleagues (Kandel et al., 1986); Kaplan and colleagues (Kaplan, 1985; Kaplan et al., 1988); Kellam and colleagues (Kellam et al., 1983); Newcomb and Bentler (1988, 1989); Pandina and colleagues (Pandina et al., 1984; Labouvie et al., in press); Pentz and colleagues (Pentz et al., 1986); and others. The following discussions draw heavily on these studies. We first review some of the literature that has focused on single risk factors; the yield of this literature is rather low, so we have been highly selective in attempting to represent it, pointing out major conclusions of studies on the role of genetic and congenital factors, personality characteristics, and socioeconomic neighborhood characteristics. We then review the results of studies on multiple risk factors that focus attention on the issue of how these risk factors interrelate.

Genetic and Congenital Predispositions

Since psychoactive drugs are chemical agents that work inside the body, it is natural to think that biological factors, including biologically heritable factors, play some part in promoting or inhibiting the onset of drug use, abuse, and dependence. The evidence for this hypothesis, however, was indirect and slender at the time of the committee's review for all drugs except alcohol. For alcohol, the heritability of some tendency—heavily modulated by environmental and developmental features—appears reasonably well established.

The evidence for biological risk factors is of two kinds. First, different strains of animal species bred for laboratory studies vary in their predilection or resistance to consuming alcohol and other drugs, and these preferences can be altered over generations through selective breeding. (These preferences can also be altered through training; trained behaviors are not, of course, genetically transmissible, although quickness in learning is.)

Second, there is evidence from behavioral-genetic and related studies with human populations. Most of this work pertains to alcoholism, although there is evidence from other pharmacogenetic and genetic epidemiological research indicating predispositions to other types of drug abuse and dependence (Institute of Medicine, 1989; Pickens and Svikis, 1988; Pickens et al., 1991). Family and twin studies suggest that there is a genetic predisposition toward one of two typical patterns of alcoholism. Children with a biological parent who has developed clinical alcoholism, even if this parent had no role whatsoever in their childrearing (e.g., children adopted at birth), are at four- to tenfold greater risk of this outcome compared with matched children whose biological parents are without a clinical history of alcoholism (Cloninger et al., 1981; Goodwin, 1983).

One index of risk that has not been well studied is the magnitude of dissonance among biological, cognitive, and behavioral spheres of functioning during the early second decade. It has been observed that girls who enter puberty early may not yet be equipped with a number of social and cognitive skills commensurate with biological maturation. They may therefore be at increased risk for a number of adverse outcomes, perhaps for as long as a decade afterward, including drug and alcohol abuse, antisocial disorder, school dropout and unplanned pregnancy (Magnussen et al., 1986). The age at menarche, as one biological marker of a host of anatomical, hormonal, and social changes, has been dropping steadily over the past 40 years, and social institutions have adjusted unevenly to these maturational developments.

Overall, the place of biological heritage and biological mediation in explaining the onset of drug use, abuse, and dependence remains uncertain. Further human population research that attends as carefully to environmental conditioning as to physiological measures is needed to evaluate the relative role of neurochemical and other biological predisposing factors. Although it is premature to recommend trials of strategies for informing people of their possible risk based on family history of drug use, further analysis of the potential risks and benefits of such advice (e.g., the risks of labeling people and reduced self-esteem versus the benefits of reduced use of drugs) is justified in anticipation of improved biological markers of risk (Bamberg et al., 1990; Becker and Janz, 1987; Bensley, 1981; Childs, 1974; Hunt et al., 1986; Khowry et al., 1985; Zylke, 1987).

Personality Characteristics

Only a small number of the many personality characteristics that have been investigated in connection with drug use have shown significant results as risk factors (Lang, 1983). Among these few characteristics, the most positive evidence has accumulated in support of a psychological construct called *sensation seeking*. In contrast, such factors as depression, suicidal thoughts, and low self-esteem, all of which seem very plausible and often serve as commonsense assumptions underlying the design of drug abuse prevention efforts, do not stand up well under empirical investigation.

Zuckerman (1979) described sensation seeking as a fundamental aspect of personality based in the neurochemistry of monamine oxidase. His four measures of sensation seeking—seeking new experiences, seeking thrills or adventure, susceptibility to boredom, and disinhibition—have been shown to correlate with a number of illicit activities, including alcohol and drug use, in adolescent and young adult populations (Bates et al., 1985; Huba et al., 1981). In studies using the Rutgers longitudinal sample, sensation seeking and negative affectivity proved to have much larger effects on drug use, both independently and interactively, than positive affectivity. Newcomb and McGee (1989), using multivariate methods to probe results with the UCLA sample, found that sensation seeking had unexpectedly complex effects, differing for males and females, with the most pronounced relation to high levels of alcohol use.

Many clinicians believe that specific emotional disorders, particularly depression and related distress, trigger or severely aggravate drug use, abuse, or dependence. The evidence in this direction is inconsistent. Kaplan (1985), Huba et al., (1986), Aneshensel and Huba (1983), and Labouvie (1986) all found that drug use is often preceded by emotional distress or depression. But the relieving effects of drug use on these states is short-lived. Newcomb and Bentler (1988) found that alcohol use over time in a general population sample of adolescents was correlated with a reduction in depression, but no such correlation emerged linking other drug use to depression or other emotional distress. Elliott and Huizinga (1984) found that emotional problems and social isolation (feelings of loneliness) were moderately correlated with the level of use of alcohol, marijuana, and other illicit drugs in a general youth population sample. Dembo and colleagues (1991) found a similar result among detainees in a juvenile detention center.

The most extreme level of depression is suicidal thinking and attempts. Suicide is the second leading cause of death among adolescents. However, drug use seems to be more a risk factor for suicide attempts than the other way around. Newcomb and Bentler (1988) reported that adolescent use of "hard" drugs (beyond alcohol and marijuana) was associated with subsequently increased suicidal thinking in young adulthood.

The belief is widely held and intuitively appealing that a strong sense of self-esteem is a protective factor and lack of it a risk factor for adolescent drug use. There is no doubt that most cases of adolescent drug abuse or dependence that come to clinical attention are individuals who are short on self-esteem. The specific notion is that individuals with low self-esteem seek drugs in order to raise it (Kaplan, 1986). Numerous preventive interventions have applied this theory by seeking to build up their participants' self-esteem, teaching them how to raise it, or expanding the opportunities for enhancing self-esteem in ways other than by taking drugs.

Despite its attractions, the evidence for the self-esteem theory is mostly not supportive. In large studies such as White et al. (1986) and Kaplan et al. (1984), very weak correlations were observed between self-esteem and drug use, and these variables paled into insignificance under further statistical manipulation. Even if self-esteem did seem to be an important risk factor for drug taking, the idea that it might be altered by any of the program measures ordinarily undertaken is problematic, denying or ignoring as it does commonly assumed determinants of self-esteem such as physical attractiveness (Simcha-Fagen et al., 1986).

In summary, the search for specific personality risk factors for illicit drug taking has been mostly disappointing. Studies on sensation seeking, an active trait, have proven more promising than those focusing on more inward-turning characteristics such as depression and self-devaluation.

Socioeconomic Factors at the Neighborhood Level

The epidemiologic evidence indicates that onset of illicit drug use occurs mainly through peer group contact and that rates of onset (as distinct from continued use) are at rather similar levels within economic and ethnic groups. We suspect that the illicit drug use and trafficking that occur in economically disadvantaged communities, which are disproportionately black, Puerto Rican, and Mexican-American, occur for many of the same reasons as in other segments of the population, but that these reasons are more intense. In the most depressed portions of these communities, there is an additional dimension associated with greater numbers of drug abusing and dependent individuals and high levels of violence: namely, for many poor, young minority men and women, illicit drug markets are key sources of employment and are perceived as a route to economic mobility. In order to be successful in selling drugs, it is necessary for these young people to encourage drug use aggressively among the most vulnerable members of the community and to be prepared to enforce and protect their transactions in an increasingly gun-ridden and anarchic environment.

As Brunswick (1988) notes in her longitudinal study of several hundred youths from central Harlem: "An often overlooked cornerstone of hard drug use among young black males is that it is not only and perhaps not primarily a consumption and/or recreational behavior. It also serves economic functions of occupation and career for this group" (see also Johnson et al., 1985; Preble and Casey, 1966; Williams and Kornblum, 1986). In a population subgroup in which employment opportunities are severely constrained, and at a life stage at which economic independence is expected and required, the drug economy is one of the relatively few high-wage options that seem wide open (Reuter et al., 1990).

It is not known with certainty what distinguishes those who sell drugs in economically disadvantaged communities from the majority of their peers in these areas who, with similarly limited opportunities, shun drug involvement, or from those in the middle who use but do not sell drugs. The perception and fact of being socially distant from mainstream opportunities, at the same time needing money in order to survive, are important. But, in every ethnic group in subcommunities dominated by drug use and sales, families are the most important social unit—particularly so given the paucity of institutional infrastructure in most economically impoverished areas. Although drug users in poor minority subcommunities are predominantly from single-parent, female-headed households, the same is true of those adolescents who do not use drugs (Fitzpatrick, 1990). Whether or not there is an intact nuclear family, the most important family inhibitions against drug use (either through predisposition or through reinforcement) may be the active involvement of multiple adults—in the immediate or extended family or even among nonfamily members—in the lives of young people who are environmentally at risk (see, for example, Kellam et al., 1983; Zimmerman and Maton, 1992).

Another unknown is how differential aspects of African-American, Puerto Rican, Mexican-American, and other cultures serve as barriers to or promoters of drug use, as mediating factors in the initiation and conduct of drug use, and potential influences on the routes by which users can become drug free. Blount and Dembo (1984) assessed levels of alcohol and marijuana use among approximately 1,000 Cuban and Puerto Rican youths in inner-city junior high schools, using questionnaires based on extensive ethnographic work in these areas, which incorporated local cultural patterns by paying particular attention to perceptions of the "toughness" and level of drug involvement in the respondents' immediate neighborhoods. The results provide a textured picture of the differing contingencies that inner-city youths confront.

Participation in street culture during leisure hours was highly correlated with marijuana use, especially in the toughest neighborhoods (Blount and Dembo, 1984). The correlation between respondent and peer group marijuana use was appreciably stronger in the tougher, more drug-involved neighborhoods. In other words, in tough neighborhoods, you are either with the pot smokers or not—it is rare to have close friends among abstainers and smokers at the same time. In contrast, alcohol use was not correlated with street culture—it cut across neighborhood differences, and the positive association between respondent and peer group alcohol use was about the same everywhere. The attitudes, peer group relations, and adult role models of nonusers, alcohol-only, and alcohol-and-marijuana users were consistently different. Beyond these differences, the need to choose starkly between friendships with tough kids—who are usually marijuana users—and friendships with nonusers was a fact of life in the toughest neighborhoods, one that youths in less combative zones—even in the inner city—could more readily finesse, and one that was not present with respect to alcohol, regardless of neighborhood.

Relationships Among Risk Factors

Young people who engage in one form of health-compromising behavior are often engaged in other problem behaviors (Jessor and Jessor, 1977). The co-occurrence of alcohol and other drug abuse with delinquency and criminal behavior is well established (Elliott et al., 1985; Hawkins et al. 1987; White, 1990). From the perspective of temporal order (and thus relevant to predispositions), the first involvement in delinquent activity usually predates illicit drug use. But findings from a number of longitudinal studies (e.g., Jones, 1968, 1971; McCord and McCord, 1962; Monnelly et al., 1983; Ricks and Berry, 1970; Robins, 1966, 1978) suggest that drug use and antisocial behavior in adolescents have similar precursors: aggressive behavior, school conduct problems, poor grades, and, less certainly, shyness, anxiety, depression, and problems in peer relationships. Early alcohol and drug use along with violent or predatory behavior and early and aggressive sexual behavior seem to be part of a general pattern of rebellion and nonconformity variously called a "deviance syndrome," "antisocial personality," "conduct disorder," or "adolescent adjustment disorder."

In an analysis based on a national longitudinal study of 11-17-year-old youths in 1976, Elliott and Morse (1987) demonstrated the interrelationship of drug use, delinquency, sexual activity, and pregnancy. They found that 71 percent of the males and 52 percent of the females who were using multiple illicit drugs were sexually active, compared with 10 percent of the males and 3 percent of the females who were not using any drugs. Along similar lines were results of a study of nearly 1,000 adolescents in Los Angeles in grades 7-9 who were resurveyed in grades 10-12 (Newcomb et al., 1986). About 51 percent of the high school age sample had used marijuana at some time. But only 22 percent of those with none of the risk factors identified (low grade point average, lack of religious participation, poor relationship with parents, early alcohol use, low self-esteem, lack of conformity, sensation seeking, perception of ease of obtaining drugs, perception of neutral or favorable norms concerning drug use) had used marijuana, compared with 94 percent of those with 7 or more risk factors. These results were consistent for all other drugs and for higher levels of consumption. About 8 percent of the sample were using marijuana on a daily basis. Of youths in the sample with zero risk factors, however, less than 1 percent were daily marijuana users; of those with 7 or more risk factors, 56 percent were daily marijuana users.

No single predisposing factor dominates these analyses; rather, movement toward drug problems seems to proceed by the accumulation of small and mutually supporting effects over time—throughout early childhood and into the adolescent window of onset. The movement is a general drift toward adolescent problem behavior of various kinds and away from prosocial pursuits. If this drift across a continuum into increasingly problematic areas is indeed the principal type of causal process predisposing toward drug use, and particularly toward the higher (and more diversified) levels of consumption that mark abuse and dependence, then a preventive approach that attends systematically to a broad range of variables across a span of childhood years would be highly attractive. It is similar in this regard to the gradual accumulation of risk for heart disease and cancer from the cumulative effects of relatively innocuous discrete acts and gradually changing behavior patterns. Risk factor research thus seems to lead fairly directly to a developmental turn.

Research Needs

The study of multiple risk factors and their interaction appears to present substantial advances over attention to single factors or limited clusters of factors. This is not to say that more tightly focused studies should not be undertaken, but that such studies are best viewed as leading toward results that can be incorporated into larger-scale multivariate studies. There are needs for refinement of risk-factor research in several directions, but one in particular deserves emphasis here: methodological investment in improving techniques of measurement, particularly of environmental factors.

A major reason for improved measurement is to avoid statistical biases (descriptive and inferential) in multivariate analyses. For example, factors such as personality traits are generally measured by multi-item scales administered to the individual and scored to identify the extent of individual variation from population parameters. In contrast, factors such as neighborhood quality, which urban researchers find can vary literally by the block in many areas, are usually measured at the level of the census tract or larger geographic swaths, using such proxies as average housing cost or population density, aggregated into quartiles, or loose "urbanicity" measures based on proximity to traditional city cores. The measurement error (in terms of an accurate index of the individual's experience) that accrues from averaging across many blocks and then assigning individuals into such large, often ill-fitting categories ensures that, even if neighborhood quality or other collective characteristics were a powerful influence on the individual's behavior, these effects would be virtually precluded from statistical detection. This measurement bias would lead to false negative or Type II errors, in contrast to the likelihood that weak but transitory effects may be detected by finely calibrated personality variables that are measured at the individual level, leading to false-positive or Type I errors.

THE DEVELOPMENTAL APPROACH

A Model of Progressive Problem Behavior

A four-stage model of behavioral problems accumulating across time, which draws together a large literature (Kumpfer, 1989), has been described by Schaps and Battistich (1991). This model suggests that socialization deficits in early childhood lead young people to affiliate with peers opposed to traditional institutions (such as school), a tendency that culminates in social alienation and trouble with the law (and other conventional institutions of society) in late adolescence and adulthood. This model parallels the logical progression of drug use to abuse to dependence, in that a relatively small proportion of youths who embark on the path of drug use continue on to dependence.

In the first stage of the model, poor parenting (or, more generally, childrearing) practices in the family or among major alternative caretakers, which are evident during the preschool years, lead to low emotional attachment to parents, resistance to parental authority, early behavioral and emotional problems, and generalized developmental immaturity (poor attention span, poor impulse control). Negative parenting practices include low levels of parental affection, lack of concern and insensitivity to the child's needs, lack of supervision, hostility, rejection, and very inconsistent or punitive discipline. If parenting practices to which the child is subject do not improve, these patterns of poor family bonding become more violent and reciprocal as the child grows beyond preschool.

Although family economic conditions do not directly determine parenting practices, high levels of stress and disorganization degrade parenting performance, and these levels of stress are more common when family economic resources are scarce and when the neighborhood environment is itself impoverished and disorganized. The effects of discrimination based on race or ethnicity add to these stressors.

In the second stage, poor socialization in the family leads to emotional and conduct problems in school grades 1-3. Peers and teachers respond antagonistically to poorly socialized behavior, and the child in turn is beset by social isolation or rejection, anxiety, insecurity, and continued conflicts with authority. The course of this second stage is obviously affected by the ability of the classroom teacher to adapt to poorly socialized children and educe not simply a modicum of compliance but rather positive bonding with the school, its staff, and other students.

In the third stage, middle to late elementary grades 3-6, persistent problems in social adaptation result in decreased learning and poor grades. Deficient academic performance in turn creates isolation from and rejection by more academically competent peers; problems in adaptation to school transform into active alienation from school. It is among these youths that the early onset of tobacco or alcohol use, and in some instances marijuana as well, will occur.

In the fourth stage, junior high school continuing on into high school, students disaffected from schooling firmly withdraw their efforts from academic or any other school-organized pursuits, become more overtly rebellious, and associate with each other in increasing opposition to academically competent and socially conventional peers, who reciprocate the hostility. An increasingly exclusive association with alienated peers intensifies into a *school-oppositional peer group* culture (Willis, 1977), characterized by expressive rejection of the conventional social norms and values, continuing academic failure, alcohol and drug use, delinquent activities, sexual behavior resulting in pregnancy, and a higher probability of early school exit.

Schools themselves unintentionally further perpetuate this "clustering" of alienated adolescents by their policies of remedial education placement and detention—activities that group these students together (Oetting and Beauvias, 1987).

Interventions that assume school-based peer ties and adult-student solidarity will not be appropriate to committed members of the school-oppositional culture. Interventions that work as a reinforcer or accelerator of antidrug trends in the school-solidary culture may have null or even rebound effects in the school-oppositional one. In most schools, oppositional norms characterize a marginalized, limited proportion of students. In some, these hold the allegiance of a large fraction or even the majority, for example, in "special schools" for disciplinary problems, schools for emotionally disturbed youths, and schools that experience drop-out rates prior to high school graduation of 50 percent or higher (Lorion et al., 1989).

The school-oppositional culture is resilient, a bed of resistance or rebellion that responds strongly to attempts to affect it; it "pushes back" in ways that rebound into the larger society. Efforts to vilify characteristic practices or rituals of oppositional groups may have the perverse effect of strengthening those practices or amplifying the groups' sense of distance and rejection. In cultures formed out of economic and normative marginalization, particularly within communities that are precariously bound to begin with, all identity appears to be formed around antimainstream attitudes; those involved, however, do in fact claim to hold many mainstream values despite some forms of denial or nonparticipation—a good example being the drug dealer who says "I'm a businessman."

Entry into the later stages of systematic, deep-seated deviance implies that earlier stages have probably occurred. But some children who become academically troubled or transfer all of their loyalty into school-oppositional culture have not experienced all of the earlier stages. School opposition may not reflect alienation from family, for example, if the school is not generally integrated into a subculture, which is evidently the case in certain Native American and Mexican-American communities in metropolitan and rural areas. Nor will all the individuals at any one stage progress to later ones. In major longitudinal studies, no more than 30-40 percent of the early elementary children who displayed behavior problems engaged in antisocial behavior, delinquency, or drug abuse in adolescence (Robins, 1978). Parenting practices can improve or deteriorate over time, as family structures change through divorce or remarriage, parents mature, marital discord emerges, etc. An unusually positive school experience may counter a poor home environment; strong academic aptitude may prevail despite conduct problems; or uncompensated learning disabilities may erode initially successful academic work and school attachment.

Taking the Model Seriously: Reforming the School

Despite the many sources of variance described above, the model of problem-behavior development has strong theoretical appeal and a variety of empirical supports. It is gaining increasing attention due to concern over the steady diminution in social attentiveness to children and a generalized social deficit in parenting, of which the more extreme cases of child abuse are only a fraction. Much has been written about the relative demise of the two-parent nuclear and the extended family (Schroeder, 1989), the disappearance of personal neighborhoods and other forms of continuous local community (Green, 1990), and the increasing separation of children and youth from adult workplaces and occupational pursuits (McMillan and Chavis, 1986). These trends have resulted in the separation of children from adults in a way that is historically unprecedented. They have also served to limit caring, stable relationships between children and adults and to deprive children of meaningful exposure to a range of adult models and situations.

It is largely through close relationships with adults—mostly in the roles of parents, relatives, and teachers—that children learn how to function as adults and develop motivation to take on adult responsibilities. As they are stripped of opportunities for such relationships, it is media portrayals to which they must increasingly turn for information about "what to become." The open, pluralistic character of American society and the great freedom that this potentially provides to select personal behavior is, in a sense, lost on children whose ideas and aspirations are increasingly encapsulated within a peer social system whose culture is heavily oriented to electronic media figures—surreal, postural, and fantastic—especially when they are antagonistic to schools and other conventional institutions.

The societal trends are pervasive, cutting across virtually all demographic categories. The observation is becoming increasingly common that vast numbers of American children are now "at risk" (see Carnegie Council on Adolescent Development, 1989; National Commission on the Role of the School and the Community in Improving Adolescent Health, 1990). There is undoubtedly variation in the degree to which children are lacking in sustained adult connections and guidance, are excluded from exposure to responsible adult roles, and are living in environments saturated with opportunities for problem behaviors. It is probable that such conditions now prevail in extreme forms for many and in milder ones for most children, and that widespread experimentation with problem behaviors, including drug abuse in one form or another, may prove endemic, even though waves of such behavior will advance and recede.

American schools have changed less in the past few generations than have the other major socializing institutions. Indeed, it appears highly problematic that schools have changed so little in the face of dramatic changes elsewhere. Most schools, rather than trying to compensate for the growing deficiencies in students' lives, are deemphasizing personal relationships between children and teachers (Carnegie Council on Adolescent Development, 1989). Instead, their focus is on rigor and efficiency, in reaction to recent concerns about academic achievement, particularly in science and mathematics. Strengthening child-adult relationships is simply not viewed as a priority in how schools are organized and how teacher time is allocated. The typical classroom is structured, impersonal, and formal (Goodlad, 1984), and students are given little opportunity to take guided responsibility for their own learning or to learn service to others.

Other school characteristics compound this problem. Curricula heavily focused on developing basic cognitive skills and acquiring facts provide students few opportunities to demonstrate mastery, to see connections with "real life," or to develop the higher-order cognitive skills and social competencies they will need to experience satisfying interpersonal relationships, to resist dysfunctional social pressures, and to take on adult roles. Most schools rely on competitive evaluation systems and pervasive use of extrinsic rewards, practices that adversely affect many children's sense of competence, self-esteem, intrinsic motivation for learning, and actual performance (Deci and Ryan, 1985).

As a result, students' motivation to learn seems to be declining; many students see classroom work as meaningless and not worth the effort to succeed (Ames, in press; Zimiles, 1986). The impersonal competitive classroom atmosphere alienates many as they progress through school, leading to negative perceptions of self-worth, reduced academic efforts, more frequent misbehavior. Schools may respond by imposing an even heavier "curriculum of control" (Knitzer et al., 1990), and the downward spiral ensues.

In recognition of these and other problems, some recent thinking in education has begun to shift toward a greater concern with developmental relevance (Katz, 1989), promotion of intrinsic motivation (Deci and Ryan, 1985; Nicholls, 1989), the active role of the learner as a "maker of meaning" (Resnick, 1989), attention to social and moral development as a legitimate aspect of the curriculum (Ryan, 1986), and the importance of whether the school is a "caring community" (Carnegie Council on Adolescent Development, 1989). Although these perspectives are gaining attention, for the most part they have not been translated into research and practical applications.

To the degree that an interaction among several influences determines the occurrence of problem behaviors (Goodstadt, 1986; Huba et al., 1980), preventive interventions should provide a set of mutually reinforcing positive influences that affect all of the relevant socializing agencies (the peer group, the family, the school, the wider social community). This is in contrast to the notion that only one or two primary variables should be addressed (e.g., lack of accurate knowledge about drugs, poor resistance or assertiveness skills, early antisocial habits of behavior; see Durlak, 1985; Klitzner et al., 1985). Of course, a multilevel intervention strategy is much more demanding than one concentrating on one or two variables.

One important strand of prevention is focused on reforming the school. This reform movement views prevention not as a circumscribed, limited-duration, add-on module of curriculum designed to contravene certain negative possibilities (Moskowitz, 1987a, 1987b) but as a comprehensive effect of an entire climate of school experience that facilitates and promotes positive, effective socialization. The content of this reform includes revision of organizational structures, classroom management practices, school policies, teacher-student relationships, and instructional approaches with the intention of fostering children's social, personal, and academic development. These reforms are intended to commence with the first school exposure in the primary grades, so that the preventive effects are fully transmitted well before the early second decade when the onset of problems such as illicit drug use—which problems are most persistent and least amenable to remedial intervention—occur.

Research Needs

Research is particularly needed on the role of school organization, environment, norms, policies, and social processes and their effects on problem behaviors such as drug and alcohol use, abuse, and dependence. The school as a social institution has received much less attention in research on drug abuse prevention than have the characteristics of individual children, their families, and their peer groups. Psychological paradigms have dominated the prevention research in drug abuse; sociological paradigms have been less influential in this as in other fields of health behavior.

Prevention research needs to be diffused across the preschool and elementary levels as well as secondary school ages; the balance of concentration has been badly off kilter in the direction of middle and junior high school cohorts, in which the unprevented problems manifest themselves. Only when research is focused on this longer period can we identify critical stages and factors of development—if there are any—for problems that persist and become increasingly serious in adolescence—and hence do a better job of selecting optimal times, types, and intensities of intervention.

SOCIAL INFLUENCE AND SOCIAL LEARNING

In Chapter 1, we reviewed evidence concerning the role of cigarette smoking as a gateway to further drug consumption. The relationship established between smoking and other drug use passes various important tests of causality: appropriate temporal ordering; a substantial level of correlation, which does not vanish under multivariate analysis; a clearly described and well-studied set of intervening mechanisms (particularly, in this instance, differential access to systems of distribution); the existence of scalable dose-response relationships; and, finally, demonstration that the relationship holds across varying population groups, such as those of differing socioeconomic status. The committee took this not as evidence that cigarette smoking inevitably *causes* drug use, but as evidence that the prevention of smoking could help forestall, if not prevent, the onset of drug use.

Even if cigarettes did not hold this special salience for the onset of illicit drug use, significant attention would have to be given to smoking in this report. For cigarette smoking, due to its well-established role in the genesis of lung cancer, heart disease, and numerous other health problems, has been subject to some of the best-known and well-documented public health promotion and disease prevention campaigns of the last 40 years (see Warner, 1977). Cigarettes were a major focus not only of mass media programs but also pioneering large-scale experiments in cardiovascular risk reduction beginning in the early 1970s (the Stanford 3-community and 5-community studies by Farquhar and associates [1990] and the North Karelia project in Finland reported by Puska and colleagues [1981; 1985]). The large-scale study of smoking reduction continues today with the city-level COMMIT and state-level ASSIST trials supported by the National Cancer Institute.

Smoking was also the focus of an influential school-based prevention program conducted and reported by Evans and colleagues (Evans and Raines, 1982), which has become the model for a succession of closely watched school-based drug abuse prevention programs organized by researchers and conducted along experimental and quasi-experimental lines in the 1980s. The national "Just Say No" campaign publicized by Nancy Reagan leaned on this line of research for its justification. Flay (1987) has defined four generations of such studies, differing in the scale of experimentation, rigor of design, and quality and intensity of measurement: (1) the early pilot studies by Evans and colleagues; (2) more extensive pilot experiments by research groups based at Stanford and Minnesota (McAlister et al., 1980); (3) substantial field experiments by the latter teams and others in Scandinavia (Puska et al., 1985) and Los Angeles (Johnson et al., 1986); and (4) long-term multisite programs such as the Waterloo trials in Canada (Flay et al., 1985), the Kansas City and Indianapolis STAR studies of the USC Mid-western Prevention Project (Pentz et al., 1989), and the RAND Corporation's Project ALERT (Ellickson and Bell, 1990). One might add to this last generation a series of more comprehensive school health curriculum evalua-tions directed not specifically at drug abuse prevention but including at least prevention of smoking onset as a dependent variable (Connell and Turner, 1985; Connell et al., 1985).

Many programs are theory based, specifying which risk factors or mediating variables they are trying to change and measuring whether these are in fact changed by program exposure. Studies of social influence intervention studies have measured changes in information, in specifically instructed interactive skills, and in normative expectations regarding alcohol, tobacco, and drug use. MacKinnon et al. (1991) analyzed the first year of the Kansas City STAR program and found that a large share of the observed desirable effects were best explained by changes in normative expectations among program-exposed youth.

The fundamental work of Evans and colleagues (Evans, 1976; Evans et al. 1978, 1981) relied heavily on McGuire's (1964) "social inoculation" and "resistance to persuasive communication" theories for background. They drew most heavily, however, on Bandura's (1977, 1982, 1986) theories of social learning and his prescriptions for enhancing perceived self-efficacy: (1) specifying very explicit and proximal goals of training—in this case, resistance skills; (2) promoting accomplishments of performance through participation and practice; (3) providing models of successful behavior—in this case, peer models; and (4) providing task-specific feedback to reinforce and validate successful performance.

The most fully developed, research-based, social-influence programs are cast from a single mold. Virtually all are based on a core of junior high or middle school classroom lessons given by regular teachers, trained "peer leaders," or specialized health educators. The curriculum runs through a sequence of modules attending to predisposing, enabling, and reinforcing factors, with central attention to the development of resistance behaviors against the initial opportunity to use drugs (tobacco, alcohol, or marijuana) in a peer group context. Ellickson et al. (1988:vi-vii) give a cogent sketch of a typical lesson plan, the 7th and 8th grade ALERT program:

> The first two lessons are intended to develop motivation to resist by sharpening students' perception of the seriousness of drug use and by revealing their personal susceptibility to the harmful effects of such use [predispositional factors]. The next three lessons focus on resistance skills—helping students to identify pressures to use drugs, counter prodrug messages and learn how to say "no" to both internal and external pressures [enabling factors]. The final three sessions reinforce the earlier content and clarify the benefits of resistance. During the eighth grade, students receive a three-session booster curriculum designed to reinforce resistance skills learned the previous year [reinforcing factors].
>
> The curriculum provides multiple opportunities for student participation— role playing, question and answer techniques, small group activities, individual and group practice in saying "no," and written exercises.

There is some diversity among social influence researchers in how narrowly or broadly the programs are defined. Pentz et al. (1989) have proposed embedding the school-based curriculum within more comprehensive school and community efforts, for example, efforts to invigorate school antidrug policies and to mobilize community-wide awareness and support. Most of the research, however, has been focused on the curriculum component. There are differences here as well concerning the degree to which there is an emphasis on building general social competence or skills (such as assertiveness) in addition to ones targeted specifically at resisting peer-stimulated drug onset. This division between targeting proximal variables that will affect drug behavior but not (according to design) much else versus generic training that may have effects in many directions is characteristic of the larger school health education field, which has moved increasingly from categorical toward comprehensive programming (Green and Iverson, 1982; Kolbe and Iverson, 1983).

Research Needs

A particular problem with social influence models is the implicit assumption that school-based influence encompasses all young people. The needs for recognition of many youths, especially economically disadvantaged children in inner cities, are not well enough served by the schools to lead them to look to schools or even to their peers within the school framework for practical or moral instruction. These youths largely define themselves by their street peer loyalties, not by school district lines. Peer influences, as defined in research literature, are too often generalized as though all adolescents were culturally homogeneous; there is not enough research that recognizes the specific features of ethnic and street culture (Becker et al., 1989).

The foundations of social influence theory were in relatively small-scale social psychological studies, and more of these are needed now to extend our understanding of influence processes. More fundamental research is needed on small groups with a variety of youth-cultural affiliations. The careful studies in the 1950s and 1960s of institutionalized street gangs, including attempts to change them, are a model worth reconsidering.

SUMMARY

Three principal approaches in drug abuse prevention research emerge from the recent past: the study of risk factors, the study of developmental sequences, and the study of social influence. It is helpful in seeing how these approaches relate to each other to note their differential emphasis on predisposing, enabling, and reinforcing elements or variables in the respective theories and methods of inquiry.

The risk factors under study include biological, personality, and socioeconomic variables. In general, under longitudinal study, risk factors seem to operate as individually small but cumulative causes of criterion behaviors. These studies generally suggest prevention strategies based on identification of the high-risk youths, those for whom many such factors apply. Studies of risk factors are hobbled by measurement deficiencies with respect to environmental variables in particular, and methodological investments and improvements in this respect are needed.

The developmental approach involves a more structured, sequential model of poor early parenting, school maladjustment, academic deficiency, and gravitation toward school-oppositional groups, which are seedbeds of illicit drug use and other disorderly and problem behaviors. This approach incorporates the general sense that there is a weakening of family bonds throughout the population and that primary schools, which may be more amenable to intervention—particularly experimental intervention—than family units, should be a key locus of study.

The study of social influences, largely in junior high school populations, has also been based on a highly structured theory derived from the concept of self-efficacy and its roots in social learning. While these theoretical foundations have been extensively researched and appear robust in many ways, there has not been enough study of the differentiated social and normative world of early adolescence. This applies particularly to the emergence and significance of norms strongly antagonistic to schools and to the perception by adolescents of prodrug or antidrug norms in their peers. These are critical reinforcing environments that may make or break intervention strategies, so it is critical to build a more systematic understanding of them.

REFERENCES

Ames, C.
    in   The enhancement of student motivation, In M.L. Maehr and D.A. Kleiber, eds.,
    press   *Advances in Motivation and Achievement*, Vol. 5. Greenwich, Conn.: JAI Press.
Aneshensel, C.S., and G.J. Huba
    1983   Depression, alcohol use, and smoking over one year: a four-wave longitudinal
              causal model. *Journal of Abnormal Psychology* 92:134-150.
Bamberg, R., R.T. Acton, J.M. Roseman, R.C.P. Go, B.O. Barger, C.J. Vanichanan, and R.B.
              Copeland
    1990   The effect of genetic risk information and health risk assessment on compliance
              with preventive behaviors. *Health Education* 21(2):26-32.
Bandura, A.
    1977   *Social Learning Theory*. Englewood Cliffs, N.J.: Prentice-Hall.
Bandura, A.
    1982   Self-efficacy mechanisms in human agency. *American Psychologist* 37:122-147.

Bandura, A.
1986   *Social Foundations of Thought and Action: A Social Cognitive Theory.* Englewood Cliffs, N.J.: Prentice-Hall.

Bates, M.E., E.W. Labouvie, and H.R. White
1985   The effect of sensation seeking needs on alcohol and marijuana use in adolescence. *Bulletin of HTE Society of Psychologists in Addictive Behaviors* 5:29-36.

Becker, M.H., and N.K. Janz
1987   On the effectiveness and utility of health hazard/health risk appraisal in clinical and non-clinical settings. *Health Services Research* 22:537-551.

Becker, S.L., J.A. Burke, R.A. Arbogast, M.J. Naughton, I. Bachman, and E. Spohn
1989   Community programs to enhance in-school anti-tobacco efforts. *Preventive Medicine* 18:221-228.

Bensley, L.B.
1981   Health risk appraisals in teaching health education in colleges and universities. *Health Education* 12:31-33.

Blount, W.R., and R. Dembo
1984   The effect of perceived neighborhood setting on self-reported tobacco, alcohol, and marijuana use among inner-city minority junior high school youth. *The International Journal of the Addictions* 19(2):175-198.

Botvin, G.J., and A. Eng
1980   A comprehensive school-based smoking prevention program. *Journal of School Health* 50:209-213.

Botvin, G.J., A. Eng, and C.L. Williams
1980   Preventing the onset of cigarette smoking through life skills training. *Preventive Medicine* 9:135-143.

Brook, J.S., D.W. Brook, A.S. Gordon, M. Whiteman, and P. Cohen
1990   The psychosocial etiology of adolescent drug use: a family interactional approach. *Genetic, Social, and General Psychology Monographs* 116:111-267.

Brunswick, A.F.
1988   Drug use and effective distress: a longitudinal study of black youth. *Advances in Adolescent Mental Health* 3:101-125.

Bry, B.H., P. McKeon, and R.J. Pandina
1982   Extent of drug use as a function of number of risk factors. *Journal of Abnormal Psychology* 91:273-279.

Carnegie Council on Adolescent Development
1989   *Turning Points: Preparing American Youth for the 21st Century.* New York: Carnegie Corporation.

Childs, B.
1974   A place for genetics in health education and vice versa. *American Journal of Human Genetics* 26:120-135.

Cloninger, C., M. Bohman, and S. Sigvardsson
1981   Inheritance of alcohol abuse: cross fostering analyses of adopted men. *Archives of General Psychiatry* 38:861-868.

Connell, D.B., and R.R. Turner
1985   The impact of instructional experience and the effects of cumulative instruction. *Journal of School Health* 55:324-331.

Connell, D.B., R.R. Turner, and E.F. Mason
1985   Summary of findings of the school health education evaluation: health promotion effectiveness, implementation and costs. *Journal of School Health* 55:316-321.

Deci, E.L., and R.M. Ryan
1985   *Intrinsic Motivation and Self-Determination in Human Behavior.* New York: Plenum.

Dembo, R., L. Williams, J. Schmeidler, E.D. Wish, A. Getreu, and E. Berry
1991   Juvenile crime and drug abuse: a prospective study of high risk youth. *Journal of Addictive Diseases* 11:5-31.
Durlak, J.A.
1985   Primary prevention of school maladjustment. *Journal of Consulting and Clinical Psychology* 53:623-620.
Ellickson, P.L., and R.M. Bell
1990   Drug prevention in junior high: a multi-site longitudinal test. *Science* 247:1299-1305.
Ellickson, P.O., R.M. Bell, M.A. Thomas, A.E. Robyn, and G.L. Zellman
1988   *Designing and Implementing Project ALERT: A Smoking and Drug Prevention Experiment.* Santa Monica, Calif.: The RAND Corporation.
Elliott, D.S., and D. Huizinga
1984   The Relationship Between Delinquent Behavior and ADM Problem Behaviors. Paper prepared for the ADAMHA/OJJDP State of the Art Research Conference on Juvenile Offenders with Serious Drug/Alcohol and Mental Health Problems, Bethesda, Md.
Elliott, D.S., and B.J. Morse
1987   Drug Use, Delinquency, and Sexual Activity. Unpublished paper.
Elliott, D.S., D. Huizinga, and S.S. Ageton
1985   *Explaining Delinquency and Drug Use.* Beverly Hills, Calif.: Sage Publications.
Elliott, D.S., D. Huizinga, and S. Menard
1989   *Multiple Problem Youth: Delinquency, Substance Use, and Mental Health Problems.* New York: Springer-Verlag.
Evans, R.I.
1976   Smoking in children: developing a social psychological strategy of deterrence. *Preventive Medicine* 5:122-127.
Evans, R.I., and B.E. Raines
1982   Control and prevention of smoking in adolescents: a psychological perspective. In T.J. Coates, A.D. Peterson, and C. Perry, eds., *Promoting Adolescent Health: A Dialog on Research and Practice.* New York: Academic Press.
Evans, R.I., R.M. Rozelle, M. Mittelmark, W.B. Hansen, A. Bane, and J. Havis
1978   Deterring the onset of smoking in children: knowledge of immediate psychological effects and coping with peer pressure, media pressure, and parent modeling. *Journal of Applied Social Psychology* 8:126-135.
Evans, R.I., R.M. Rozelle, S.E. Maxwell, B.E. Raines, C.A. Dill, T.J. Guthrie, A.H. Henderson, and P.C. Hill
1981   Social modeling films to deter smoking in adolescents: results of a three-year field investigation. *Journal of Applied Psychology* 66:399-414.
Farquhar, J.W., S.P. Fortmann, J.A. Flora, C.B. Taylor, W.L. Haskell, P.T. Williams, N. Maccoby, and P.D. Wood
1990   Effects of community-wide education on cardiovascular disease risk factors—the Stanford 5-city Project. *Journal of the American Medical Association* 264:359-365.
Fitzpatrick, J.
1990   Drugs and Puerto Ricans in New York City. Pp. 103-126 in R. Glick and J. Moore, eds., *Drugs in Hispanic Communities.* New Brunswick, N.J.: Rutgers University.
Flay, B.R.
1987   Social psychological approaches to smoking prevention: review and recommendations. Pp. 121-180 in *Advances in Health Education and Promotion*, Vol. 2. Greenwich, Conn.: JAI Press Inc.

Flay, B.R., K.K. Ryan, J.A. Best, K.S. Brown, M.W. Kersell, J.R. d'Avernas, and M.P. Zanna
    1985   Are social psychological smoking prevention programs effective? The Waterloo
            study. *Journal of Behavioral Medicine* 8:37-59.
Goodlad, J.I.
    1984   *A Place Called School.* New York: McGraw-Hill.
Goodstadt, M.S.
    1986   School-based drug education in North America: what is wrong? What can be
            done? *Journal of School Health* 56:278-281.
Goodwin, D.
    1983   Alcoholism. Pp. 195-213 in R. Tarter, ed., *The Child at Psychiatric Risk.* New
            York: Oxford University Press.
Gottlieb, N.H., and L.W. Green
    1987   Ethnicity and lifestyle health risk: some possible mechanisms. *American Journal
            of Health Promotion* 2:37-45.
Green, L.W.
    1990   The revival of community and the public obligation of academic health centers.
            Pp. 148-164 in R. Bulger, R.E. Bulger, and S. Reiser, eds., *The Role of the Aca-
            demic Health Center in Humanizing Medicine.* Ames, Iowa: University of Iowa
            Press.
Green, L.W., and D.C. Iverson
    1982   School health education. *Annual Review of Public Health* 3:321-338.
Green, L.W., and M.W. Kreuter
    1991   *Health Promotion Planning: An Educational and Environmental Approach.* Palo
            Alto, Calif.: Mayfield.
Hawkins, J.D., D.M. Lishner, and R.F. Catalano
    1987   Schooling and delinquency. In E.H. Johnson, ed., *Handbook on Crime and Delin-
            quency Prevention.* Westport, Conn.: Greenwood Press.
Heckler, M.
    1985   *Report of the Secretary's Task Force on Black and Minority Health.* Washington,
            D.C.: U.S. Department of Health and Human Services.
Huba, G.J., J.A. Wingard, and P.M. Bentler
    1980   Applications of a theory of drug use to prevention programs. *Journal of Drug
            Education* 10:25-38.
Huba, G.J., J.A. Wingard, and P.M. Bentler
    1981   A comparison of two latent causal variable models for adolescent drug use. *Jour-
            nal of Personality and Social Psychology* 40:180-193.
Huba, G.J., M.D. Newcomb, and P.M. Bentler
    1986   Adverse drug experience and drug use behaviors: a one-year longitudinal study of
            adolescents. *Journal of Pediatric Psychology* 11:203-219.
Hunt, S.C., R.R. Williams, and K.K. Barlow
    1986   A comparison of positive family history definitions for defining risk of future
            disease. *Journal of Chronic Diseases* 39:809-821.
Institute of Medicine
    1989   *Prevention and Treatment of Alcohol Problems: Research Opportunities.* Com-
            mittee to Identify Research Opportunities in the Prevention and Treatment of Al-
            cohol-Related Problems. Washington, D.C.: National Academy Press.
Jacob, J.
    1987   Black America, 1986: an overview. In *The State of Black America.* New York:
            National Urban League.
Jessor, R., and S.L. Jessor
    1977   *Problem Behavior and Psychosocial Development: A Longitudinal Study of Youth.*
            New York: Academic Press.

Jessor, R., J.E. Donovan, and F.M. Costa
1992   *Beyond Adolescence: Problem Behavior and Young Adult Development.* New York: Academic Press.

Johnson, B.D., P.J. Goldstein, E. Preble, J. Schmeidler, D.S. Lipton, B. Spunt, and T. Miller
1985   *Taking Care of Business: The Economics of Crime by Heroin Abusers.* Lexington, Mass.: Lexington Books.

Johnson, C.A., W.B. Hansen, L.M. Collins, and J.W. Graham
1986   High-school smoking prevention: results of a three-year longitudinal study. *Journal of Behavioral Medicine* 9(5):439-452.

Jones, M.C.
1968   Personality correlates and antecedents of drinking patterns in adult males. *Journal of Consulting and Clinical Psychology* 32:2-12.

Jones, M.C.
1971   Personality antecedents and correlates of drinking patterns in women. *Journal of Consulting and Clinical Psychology* 36:61-69.

Kandel, D.B., O. Simcha-Fagan, and M. Davies
1986   Risk factors for delinquency and illicit drug use from adolescence to young adulthood. *Journal of Drug Issues* 16:67-90.

Kaplan, H.B.
1985   Testing a general theory of drug abuse and other deviant adaptations. *Journal of Drug Issues* 15:477-492.

Kaplan, H.B.
1986   *Social Psychology Self-Referrent Behavior.* New York: Plenum.

Kaplan, H.B., S.S. Martin, and C. Robbins
1984   Pathways to adolescent drug use: self-derogation, peer influence, weakening of social controls, and early substance use. *Journal of Health and Social Behavior* 25:270-289.

Kaplan, H.B., R.J. Johnson, and C.A. Bailey
1988   Explaining adolescent drug use: an elaboration strategy for structural equation modeling. *Psychiatry* 51:142-163.

Katz, L.G.
1989   *Engaging Children's Minds: The Project Approach.* Norwood, N.J.: Ablex.

Kellam, S.G., C.H. Brown, B.R. Rubin, and M.E. Ensminger
1983   Paths leading to teenage psychiatric symptoms and substance abuse: developmental epidemiological studies in Woodlawn. In. S.B. Guze, F.J. Earls, and J.E. Barrett, eds., *Childhood Psychopathology and Development.* Vienna, Va.: Center for Advanced Health Studies.

Khowry, M.J., C.A. Newill, and G.A. Chase
1985   Epidemiological evaluation of screening for risk factors: application to genetic screening. *American Journal of Public Health* 75:1204-1208.

Klitzner, M., M. Blasinsky, K. Marshall, and U. Paquet
1985   *Determinants of Youth Attitudes and Skills Towards Which Drinking/Driving Prevention Programs Should be Directed,* Vol. 1. Report No. DOT HS 806-903. Springfield, Va.: National Technical Information Service.

Knitzer, J., Z. Steinberg, and B. Fleish
1990   *At the Schoolhouse Door: An Examination of Programs and Policies for Children with Behavioral and Emotional Problems.* New York: Bank Street College of Education.

Kolbe, L.J., and D.C. Iverson
1983   Integrating school and community efforts to promote health: strategies, policies and methods. *Hygie: International Journal of Health Education* 3:40-47.

Kumpfer, K.L.
  1989   Effective Parenting Strategies for High Risk Youth and Families: Literature Re-
          view. Social Research Institute, Graduate School of Social Work, University of
          Utah.
Labouvie, E.W.
  1986   Alcohol and marijuana use in relation to adolescent stress. *International Journal
          of the Addictions* 21:333-345.
Labouvie, E.W., R.J. Pandina, and V. Johnson
  in press Developmental trajectories of substance use in adolescence: differences and pre-
          dictors. *International Journal of Behavioral Development.*
Lang, A.R.
  1983   Addictive personality: a viable construct? Pp. 157-236 in P.K. Levison, D.R.
          Gerstein, and D.R. Maloff, eds., *Commonalities in Substance Abuse and Habitual
          Behavior.* Lexington, Mass.: D.C. Health and Company.
Lorion, R.P., D. Bussell, and R. Goldberg
  1989   *Identification and Assessment of Youths at High Risk of Substance Abuse.* Rockville,
          Md.: Office of Substance Abuse Prevention.
MacKinnon, D.P., C.A. Johnson, M.A. Pentz, J.H. Dwyer, W.B. Hanson, B.R. Flay, and E.Y.I.
          Ward
  1991   Mediating mechanisms in a school-based drug prevention program: first-year
          effects of the Midwestern Prevention Project. *Health Psychology* 10(3):164-172.
Magnussen, D., H. Statin, and V. Allen
  1986   Differential maturation among girls and its relation to social adjustment: a longi-
          tudinal perspective. In P. Baltes, D. Featherman, and R. Lerner, eds., *Life Span
          Development and Behavior.* Hillsdale, N.J.: Erlbaum.
McAlister, A.L., C. Perry, J. Killen, L.A. Slinkard, and N. Maccoby
  1980   Pilot study of smoking, alcohol, and drug abuse prevention. *American Journal of
          Public Health* 70-719-721.
McCord, W., and J. McCord
  1962   A longitudinal study of the personality of alcoholics. In D.J. Pittman and C.R.
          Snyder, eds., *Society, Culture, and Drinking Patterns.* New York: Wiley.
McGuire, W.J.
  1964   Inducing resistance to persuasion. In L. Berkowitz, ed., *Advances in Experimental
          Social Psychology,* Vol. 1. New York: Academic Press.
McMillan, D.W., and D.M. Chavis
  1986   Sense of community: a definition and theory. *Journal of Community Psychology*
          14:6-23.
Monnelly, E.P., E.M. Hartl, and R. Elderkin
  1983   Constitutional factors predictive of alcoholism in a follow-up of delinquent boys.
          Journal of Studies on Alcohol 44:530-537.
Moskowitz, J.M.
  1987a   *The Primary Prevention of Alcohol Problems: A Critical Review of the Research
          Literature.* Berkeley, Calif.: Prevention Research Center.
Moskowitz, J.M.
  1987b   *School Drug and Alcohol Policy: A Preliminary Model Relating Implementation
          to School Problems.* Berkeley, Calif.: Prevention Research Center.
National Commission on the Role of the School and the Community in Improving Adolescent
          Health
  1990   *Code Blue: Uniting for Healthier Youth.* Alexandria, Va.: National Association
          of State Boards of Education, and Chicago, Ill.: American Medical Association.
Newcomb, M.D., and P.M. Bentler
  1988   *Consequences of Adolescent Drug Use.* Beverly Hills, Calif.: Sage Publications.

Newcomb, M.D., and P.M. Bentler
1989   Substance use and abuse among children and teenagers. *American Psychologist* 44:242-248.

Newcomb, M.D., and L. McGee
1989   Alcohol use and other delinquent behaviors: a one-year longitudinal analysis controlling for sensation-seeking. *Criminal Justice Behavior* 16:345-369.

Newcomb, M.D., E. Maddahian, and P.M. Bentler
1986   Risk factors for drug use among adolescents: concurrent and longitudinal analysis. *American Journal of Public Health* 76(5):525-531.

Newcomb, M.D., E. Maddahian, R. Skager, and P.M. Bentler
1987   Substance abuse and psychosocial risk factors among teenagers: associations with sex, age, ethnicity, and type of school. *American Journal of Drug and Alcohol Abuse* 13(4):413-433.

Nicholls, J.G.
1989   *The Competitive Ethos and Democratic Education.* Cambridge, Mass.: Harvard University Press.

Oetting, E.R., and F. Beauvais
1987   Common elements in youth drug abuse: peer clusters and other psychosocial factors. *Journal of Drug Issues* (Spring):133-151.

Pandina, R.J., E.W. Labouvie, and H.R. White
1984   Potential contributions of the life span developmental approach to the study of adolescent alcohol and drug use. *Journal of Drug Issues* 14:253-270.

Pentz, M.A., C. Cormack, B. Flay, W.B. Hansen, and C.A. Johnson
1986   Balancing program and research integrity in community drug abuse prevention: project STAR approach. *Journal of School Health* 56:389-393.

Pentz, M.A., J.H. Dwyer, D.P. MacKinnon, B.R. Flay, W.B. Hansen, E.Y.I. Wang, and C.A. Johnson
1989   A multi-community trial for primary prevention of adolescent drug abuse: effects on drug use prevalence. *Journal of the American Medical Association* 261:3259-3266.

Pickens, R., and D. Svikis, eds.
1988   *Biological Vulnerability to Drug Abuse.* NIDA Research Monograph 89. Rockville, Md.: National Institute on Drug Abuse.

Pickens, R.W., D.S. Svikis, M. McGue, D.T. Lykken, L.L. Heston, and P.J. Clayton
1991   Heterogeneity in the inheritance of alcoholism. A study of male and female twins. *Archives of General Psychiatry* 48(1):19-28.

Preble E., and J.J. Casey
1966   Taking care of business: the heroin user's life on the street. *International Journal of the Addictions* 4:1-24.

Puska, P., A. McAlister, J. Pekkola, and K. Koskela
1981   Television in health promotion: evaluation of a national programme in Finland. *International Journal of Health Education* 24:2-14.

Puska, P., A. Nissinen, J. Tuomilehto, J.T. Salonen, K. Koskela, A. McAlister, T.E. Kottke, N. Maccoby, and J.W. Farquhar
1985   The community-based strategy to prevent coronary heart disease: conclusions from the ten years of the North Karelia Project. *Annual Review of Public Health* 6:147-193.

Rennert, M.P., M.J. Telch, J.W. Farquhar, and J.D. Killen
1986   Disease and risk factor clustering in the United States: the implications for public health policy. In *Integration of Risk Factor Interventions: Two Reports to the Office of Disease Prevention and Health Promotion.* Washington, D.C.: U.S. Department of Health and Human Services.

Resnick, L.B., ed.
   1989   *Knowing, Learning, and Instruction: Essays in Honor of Robert Glaser.* Hillsdale,
          N.J.: Lawrence Erlbaum.
Reuter, P., R. MacCoun, and P. Murphy
   1990   *Money from Crime. A Study of the Economics of Drug Dealing in Washington,
          D.C.* Publication R-3894-RF. Santa Monica, Calif.: The Rand Corporation.
Ricks, D., and J.C. Berry
   1970   Family and symptom patterns that precede schizonphrenia. In M. Roff and D.F.
          Hicks, eds., *Life History Research in Psychopathology.* Minneapolis, Minn.: Uni-
          versity of Minnesota Press.
Robins, L.N.
   1966   *Deviant Children Grown Up: A Sociological and Psychiatric Study of Sociopathic
          Personality.* Baltimore, Md.: Williams & Wilkins.
Robins, L.N.
   1978   Sturdy childhood predictors of adult antisocial behavior: replications from longi-
          tudinal studies. *Psychological Medicine* 8:611-622.
Ryan, K.
   1986   The new moral education. *Phi Delta Kappan* (November):228-233.
Schaps, E., and V. Battistich
   1991   Chapter in E. Goplerud, ed., *A Practical Guide to Substance Abuse Prevention in
          Adolescent.* OSAP Prevention Monograph 8. DHHS Publ No. (ADM) 91-1725.
          Washington, D.C.: U.S. Government Printing Office.
Schinke, S.P.
   1982   A school-based model for teenage pregnancy prevention. *Social Work Education*
          4:32-42.
Schinke, S.P., and L.D. Gilchrest
   1977   Adolescent pregnancy: an interpersonal skill training approach to prevention.
          Social Work in Health Care 3:159-167.
Schroeder, P.
   1989   *Champion of the Great American Family.* New York: Random House.
Simcha-Fagen, O., J.C. Gersten, and T.S. Langer
   1986   Early precursors and concurrent correlates of patterns of illicit drug use in adoles-
          cents. *Journal of Drug Issues* 16(1):7-28.
Thomas, S.B.
   1990   Social change theory: applications to community health. Pp. 45-65 in N. Bracht,
          ed., *Health Promotion at the Community Level.* Newbury Park, Calif.: Sage
          Publications.
Warner, K.E.
   1977   The effects of the anti-smoking campaign on cigarette consumption. *American
          Journal of Public Health* 67(7):645-650.
White, H.R.
   1990   The drug use-delinquency nexus in adolescence. In R. Weisheit, ed., *Drugs, Crime
          and the Criminal Justice System.* Champaign, Ill.: Anderson.
White, H.R., V. Johnson, and A. Horowitz
   1986   An application of three deviance theories to adolescent substance use. *Interna-
          tional Journal of the Addictions* 21(3):347-366.
Williams, T.M., and W. Kornblum
   1986   *Growing Up Poor.* Lexington, Mass.: Lexington Books.
Willis, P.
   1977   *Learning to Labor: How Working Class Kids Get Working Class Jobs.* New
          York: Columbia University Press.

Zimiles, H.
    1986   The changing American child: the perspective of educators. Pp. 61-84 in T.M. Tomlinson and H.J. Walberg, eds., *Academic Work and Educational Excellence.* MSSE Yearbook. Berkeley, Calif.: McCutcheon Publishing.

Zimmerman, M.A., and K.I. Maton
    1992   Lifestyle and substance use among male African-American urban adolescents: a cluster analytic approach. *American Journal of Community Psychology* 20:121-138.

Zuckerman, M.
    1979   *Sensation Seeking: Beyond the Optimal Level of Arousal.* Hillsdale, N.J.: Erlbaum.

Zylke, J.
    1987   Once identified, will high-risk families make lifestyle changes, lower coronary disease rate? Medical News and Perspective. *Journal of the American Medical Association* 258(4):

3

Evaluating Prevention
Program Effects

As we have seen, the theoretical foundations for prevention are based on three principal approaches: (1) the risk factor approach, implemented mainly in the primary grades to affect predisposing factors; (2) the developmental approach, which concentrates on the socially reinforcing properties of classrooms and family environments; and (3) the social learning approach, working in junior high and middle schools mainly to alter enabling factors, such as skills and motivation to resist media and peer influence. All three approaches use the school as the basic vehicle through which prevention efforts flow, although the stronger examples of each type of intervention recognize and seek to make positive use of the fact that schools exist within the context of family and community.

There is a related movement toward the use of mass communications media as an educational channel. Much of the theoretical foundation for social influence approaches is transferable to mass media, although communications experts view the media fundamentally as a supplemental or amplifying rather than the primary carrier of persuasive communications regarding health-related behavior.

The empirical research picture is not as tidy as the theoretical concepts. For one thing, differences that are sharp and clear in theoretical abstraction become blurred in the details of application. Most actual school-based prevention curricula, of whatever theoretical inspiration, include a number of the following components:

- *Technical information* about drugs and the consequences of use,
- Instruction on techniques for *making decisions* about drug use,
- *Clarification of values* to help put decisions about drug use in perspective,
- Instruction in *stress management* techniques,
- Exercises to enhance *self-esteem*,
- Social learning to enhance *self-efficacy,*
- Instruction in *setting goals* and working to implement them,
- *Life skills training* to assist students in resisting drug use,
- *Resistance skills training* to help students resist pressures, direct and indirect, to use drugs,
- Making a *pledge* publicly not to use drugs,
- Instruction in how to *set norms* for one's age-graded peers and self,
- Instruction in how to provide *assistance* to one's peers, and
- Identification of and encouragement to seek *alternatives* to drug use.

The empirical challenge has been to sort out the critical elements from the adventitious ones, find the best time to begin intervening, select the optimal programmatic sequence and emphasis, identify the most conducive agents of transmission, and divine the most effective ways to prepare those agents for the task.

The prevention research field is substantial enough, and of long enough standing, that a number of large-scale, meticulously conducted research evaluations of preventive interventions have been completed; numerous research reviews and collections of reviews have been published (see, for example, Goplerud, 1991; Bell and Battjes, 1987; Kumpfer, 1987). Several well-defined prevention programs have been very widely disseminated. But for various reasons, the transitions from publication of major results, to compilation of definitive reviews, to wide dissemination of practices have been less than ideal. Indeed, reading the prevention research literature brings to mind the Cheshire cat in Lewis Carroll's Wonderland: lines of work seem to resolve into vivid conclusions, which then fade away in a few critical turns of the page. The will to believe on the part of implementers and program sponsors alike seems stronger than the evidence supports.

With this forewarning, we begin the chapter by recounting widely cited recent meta-analyses of research findings on preventive interventions. To give more concrete meaning than we think can yet be gained from these synthetic reviews, we then analyze (1) a series of curricula that use cognitive and behavioral approaches in relatively limited-scale experimental interventions; (2) completed large-scale experimental studies using social influence programming; (3) prominent work now in progress probing social influence and developmental interventions; and (4) the special role of mass media as channels for prevention communications.

META-ANALYSES OF PREVENTION INTERVENTIONS

Meta-analysis refers to techniques developed by behavioral statisticians for quantitatively integrating the findings from various studies. These techniques have been described and debated in a number of recent books (e.g., Wachter and Straf, 1990) and widely used in the past decade. As Bangert-Drowns (1988:245), one of the authors reviewed below, points out, meta-analysis has two potentially major advantages over more traditional narrative reviews of the scientific literature. First, it adheres to a precisely defined metric of outcome that is comparable across studies: the intervention's *effect size*, defined as the difference between the average (mean) scores on an outcome measure of the experimental and control groups, divided by their standard deviation. Second, meta-analysis uses reproducible statistical tests to examine relations between effect sizes and characteristics of the studies being reviewed.

Two types of meta-analysis have been applied to interventions to prevent drug abuse. Tobler (1986) first employed "classic" meta-analysis (Glass et al., 1981). This method sweeps together methodologically loose as well as rigorous studies, on the grounds that evaluations of methodological strength differ, and even weak studies contain some increments of information. It treats separately each of the different numbers of outcome items collected in different studies, thus allowing some studies disproportionate weight. Bangert-Drowns (1988) employed "study effect" meta-analysis to examine school-based substance abuse education. The advantage of the study-effect approach is that it is more selective, excluding studies with serious methodological flaws, and it weights each study equally when average effect sizes are calculated. In a reanalysis, Tobler (1989) applied the more restrictive inclusion criteria and weighting used by Bangert-Drowns and then extended the new analysis by focusing on characteristics of the 10 most effective programs.

Tobler I

Tobler (1986, 1989) included 143 programs in her first widely cited meta-analysis. Four criteria were used to include a program in the meta-analysis:

- Use of quantitative outcome measures including mediating variables;
- Presence of control or comparison groups (however, in many cases these were supplied by Tobler post hoc);
- Students in grades 6-12 as recipients of intervention;
- Prevention as a goal of the intervention (i.e., assisting young people in developing attitudes, values, behavior, and skills that may reduce the likelihood of drug use).

Each program was coded for 17 different content items, which were then mapped into five program types:

• Knowledge-only, meaning purely informational programs about drug effects;
• Affective-only, meaning largely nondrug-specific curricula to enhance self-esteem or general competency skills (see further discussion below);
• Knowledge-plus-affective;
• Peer programs (which means that some program element focuses on peer interaction, either as a teaching method or as a transmitter of drug behavior—this does not necessarily mean training in peer resistance skills); and
• Alternatives, generally meaning that the subjects were treated outside a conventional school environment.

In all, 63 variables (e.g., outcome measures, client characteristics, methodological issues, program implementation, etc.) that could affect program success were coded. Tobler estimated effect sizes for program success based on outcome variables for drug knowledge; drug attitudes and values; behavioral skills (i.e., decision making, assertiveness, refusal, etc.), in terms of learning the skills and, separately, reporting instances of using them; and self-reported drug use.

Tobler (1986) found that the average effect size for change in knowledge (0.52) was nearly double the effect for desired change in nondrug behaviors (0.27), skills development (0.26), and self-reported drug use (0.24). The effect size for attitudinal change was the lowest among the outcomes assessed (0.18). Knowledge-only programs had measurable effects on knowledge but negligible effects on attitudes and self-reported drug use. Affective-only programs were, in Tobler's analysis, ineffective across all outcome measures. Knowledge-plus-affective programs had a very modest average effect size on drug use (0.15). Peer programs had the most marked effect on self-reported drug use (0.40). Alternative programs, which were highly intensive and targeted on high-risk adolescents, were midway between.

Tobler's analysis suggests that a significant effect on drug knowledge and attitudes can occur without significant parallel changes in drug use. The analysis also suggests that there are no significant differences in drug use outcome effects between urban and suburban populations and between junior and senior high students.

Tobler II

Tobler's original report was critically reviewed by Bangert-Drowns (1988). He noted that an unreported number of the evaluations included in Tobler's analysis were not located in the peer-reviewed literature and, for this and other reasons, there were far too many methodologically weak reports in the pool of studies analyzed. Moreover, he noted that an unspecified number of the studies did not include sufficient information to calculate effect sizes, which had led Tobler to improvise various unspecified imputation procedures. Finally, he noted that the overall results gave very disproportionate weight to a small group of studies with large numbers of outcome measures. (Note: this is also problematic from a statistical significance testing standpoint insofar as the samples are not independent.)

Tobler (1989) subsequently reanalyzed 91 of the 143 prevention intervention programs included in the original meta-analysis. The weakest studies were evidently excluded. This new analysis was based solely on the self-reported drug use outcome and computed only one effect size for each program. The effect sizes for knowledge-only, affective-only, and knowledge-plus-affective programs were all insignificant at 0.07 or less. The effect size on drug use outcome for peer programs was 0.42; for alternatives it was 0.20. These results were quite similar to those originally reported.

Tobler achieved further specification by focusing on the "top-10" (highest effect sizes) peer programs. Tobler found certain commonalities here, in particular an emphatic focus on group interaction and delivery of the intervention by mental health professionals or counselors rather than regular teachers or peer leaders. The most successful programs for those of junior high age stressed the acquisition of skills, particularly refusal skills, although there was evidence of efficacy for broad-spectrum (decision making, competency, life) skills as well. The top peer programs among those of high school age featured well-structured group discussions that maintained an emphasis on drugs. Tobler notes that individual sessions often augmented the group sessions.

Based on these results of scrutinizing the top 10, Tobler reanalyzed the data from the 91 programs and found that overall effect sizes for mental health professionals or counselors were at least twice the effect size for health education specialists, peer leaders, teachers, college students/others, and a combination of mental health professionals or counselors and teachers. Tobler (1989:19) noted: "The success of the peer programs is not dependent on the leader but is enhanced by the presenter. . . . Mental health professionals or counselors were represented almost entirely in the peer strategies. This combination produced the highest average effect size (0.80). When peer leaders or teachers were used in the peer strategies, their average effect sizes were equivalent (0.31)."

As clear as these results appear, direct scrutiny of the top-10 programs yields ambiguities and obstacles to generalization that neither Bangert-Drowns's nor Tobler's reanalysis addresses. One cardinal point is that Tobler's generic use of the term *drug* includes cigarettes and that 4 of the top-10 peer programs (and an uncertain number of others in the sample) focused *exclu-*

sively on cigarettes; only 3 of the 10 included measures of alcohol, marijuana, or other drugs. Half of the top 10 did not use an experimental design involving random assignment. Just 2 of the 10 studies drew representative samples of students experimentally assigned to treatment and control conditions, and in both of those studies the interventions (and outcomes reported) are specifically on cigarette smoking. In addition, program subjects were not generally followed up for long; only two had a follow-up period beyond 1 year. Despite Tobler's selectivity, the general methodological rigor and relevance of the studies included remains low. Although this would not in itself invalidate the results, a closer look at a handful of the top-10 programs stipulated by Tobler, those available in peer-reviewed venues and not restricted to cigarette smoking, provides a revealing perspective on the meta-analytic results.

One of these programs was reported by Sorensen and Jaffe (1975). It involved a total of 10 adolescents who were self-recruited to a 14-week, once-a-week "drug group" organized by a paraprofessional staff member in a storefront community youth center. Four recruits stopped participating after one or two sessions (three after a confrontation over coming to group meetings while intoxicated or in an otherwise disruptive condition); these four were used as the control group. The other six participants reported lifetime use of 9 drugs, while early departees averaged 14 drugs. These results yield an effect size of 0.71; they were, however, posttest data. No pretest data had been collected to ascertain whether control and treatment groups had different drug experiences even before the intervention, which the reasons given for the creation of the "dropout" control group certainly suggest.

In a second top-10 program, Wunderlich et al. (1974) reported on a procedure instituted in a juvenile court, in which short-term group therapy was prescribed for adolescents and their parents. The treated group of 100 parent-child cases comprised juvenile drug offenders 14-19 years old (average age 16.6), three-fourths of whom had been detained specifically on drug charges; 85 percent of their parents participated in 12-week parent groups (which were separate from those for the adolescents). The 100 comparison cases were juvenile offenders 9-18 years old (average age 15), 62 percent of whom had been detained for *non*drug-related felony offenses and 33 percent for the status offense "in need of supervision." All of the comparison group were referred to detention centers, forestry camps, or juvenile services probation. At 2-year follow-up, the comparison group (although nearly two grades younger) had left school more often (25 versus 15), been rearrested more often on nondrug offenses (41 versus 11), and had more drug rearrests (3 versus 2)—the last statistic yielding an effect size of 0.62.

In Tobler's third top-10 study, Chambers and Morehouse (1983:84-85) reported on a school-based student assistance program in which counse-

lors with master's degrees conducted individual, family, and group sessions for students. The program was publicized by counselor presentations in classrooms and letters sent home. According to the authors, "Except for students referred . . . because they were caught using alcohol or
drugs, participation is voluntary." About 70 percent of the students in the
program were classified as alcohol or drug abusers. How many of these
were mandatory referrals is unclear. Details of the evaluation procedure
are quite sketchy in the published report, and it is not clear what comprised a control group. Based presumably on unpublished data, Tobler
calculated an effect size of 0.94.

The fourth top-10 study was the only one of the four employing a
persuasively equivalent control group of reasonable size against which the
program effect size was inferred, and it was the only one using a sample of
students generalizable to most school settings (although not to the general
population of students). In this study, Horan and Williams (1982) reported
an experiment in which the least assertive one-third of girls and boys, respectively, in an 8th grade cohort were randomly assigned to three conditions: active treatment, "placebo" sessions (both types administered by
master's-level counselors), or no treatment. The students were tested just
prior to the intervention, immediately after the intervention, and again at a
3-year follow-up. The active treatment consisted of five 45-minute sessions
of assertion training over a 2-week period, each session involving three new
exercises (one of which was a peer-pressure-to-use-drugs type of stimulus)
and live modeling, role-playing, and correction of the assertive response.
The placebo sessions were comprised of discussions of assertiveness, peer
pressure, and drug use—but no modeling or role-playing.

There were no pre-post assertiveness effects in the placebo or control
groups, and no 3-year differences between placebo and controls in their use
of alcohol and marijuana or hard drugs. The active training group, however, gained significantly in pre-post assertiveness, and at 3-year follow-up
they reported three times as many total refusals and one-third as many total
episodes of using drugs; however, the many zero reports and high variance
in quantities marginalized the statistical significance of these results.

In summary, of the four top-10 peer programs reported in accessible,
refereed publications, only the one (Horan and Williams) engenders scientific confidence on the basis of a sound design—and here, the result for
which effect size was calculated was statistically suspect. Even more trouble-
some than the prevailing methodological defects is the fact that these interventions are not, by and large, drug prevention programs as the term is
generally understood. Admission to three of the four programs just reviewed required substantial levels of drug-related problems to begin with;
even the fourth program was quite selective, excluding two-thirds of students. Calling these interventions prevention rather than treatment or reha-

bilitation is difficult to justify. The fact that counseling professionals produced better results would certainly be expected if the programs were in fact therapeutic rather than prophylactic interventions.

Tobler's results in favor of peer programs—that is, interventions referring to peer interaction as a teaching or therapeutic method—may be considered suggestive to the degree that where there is smoke, even smoke amplified by mirrors, there may be fire. There is certainly a marked contrast between the positive peer results and the uniformly negative results found with three other types of interventions. Nevertheless, when closely examined, the fruits of Tobler's meta-analysis can be considered imaginative and provocative but hardly persuasive concerning the question of how effective *prevention* programs may be.

Other Meta-Analyses

Bangert-Drowns studied a selection of educational programs much more tightly screened than Tobler's. He limited the analysis to studies meeting the following stringent criteria: the programs had to be conducted in schools with "traditional students"; tobacco-only programs were excluded; a no-treatment control had to be used that was shown not to be significantly different before treatment from the experimental group; and the original data had to be reported in sufficient detail to permit unambiguous calculation of effect sizes.

Under these selection criteria, only 33 programs were admitted to the meta-analysis. Most were knowledge-only or knowledge-plus-affective programs, in Tobler's terms, and most used teachers to deliver the intervention. In all, 4 were in elementary schools, 12 in junior high or middle schools, and 17 in high school or college. Slightly over half the interventions focused exclusively on alcohol education, and half were of 5 weeks' duration or less. The evaluations employed three outcome criteria: knowledge about substances (alcohol or drugs); attitudes toward substances, their use, and abuse; and behavior with regard to substances. Of them, 26 evaluations measured knowledge, 18 measured attitudes, and 14 measured behavior; only 3 studies measured all three criteria (Bangert-Drowns, 1988).

Effects on knowledge were highest (average effect size 0.76), effects on attitudes were lower (0.34), and effects on behavior were lowest (0.12), not differing significantly from zero. No identified study feature had a consistent differential effect on knowledge. However, two program features differentially affected attitudinal results: the mode of delivery, with lecture-only as the weakest mode, and the use of peer leaders, which had significantly higher average effects in the desired direction compared with adult-led conditions, a result differing from Tobler's. Two study features reliably related to behavioral outcomes were the year of publication (the more recent the techniques, the higher the effects) and whether the students volunteered rather than being forced to participate (volunteers had higher effects).

Bangert-Drowns's sample of evaluations were skewed toward higher grades, toward an alcohol focus, and toward programs of very short duration compared with Tobler's selections. Since only a handful of the evaluations included knowledge, attitude, and behavior in the same design, conclusions about the relative effect sizes must be viewed with caution. Bangert-Drowns's exclusion of studies with significant pretreatment differences between experimental and control groups does not clarify what constituted significant initial nonequivalence—in particular, whether statistical controls over initial conditions were accepted.

Another consideration of the comparison of methods using meta-analysis is whether the grouping of studies in each category of intervention method (e.g., cognitive, cognitive-plus-affective) constituted a homogeneous set as measured by the pretest or posttest effect sizes. If not, those studies with extreme effect sizes (outliers) should be removed from the group comparison.

Bruvold and Rundall (1988) published a meta-analysis and theoretical review of 19 school-based tobacco- and alcohol-oriented intervention studies. The 19 studies all utilized a control or comparison group and met 5 design criteria. The analysis contrasted the "rational" prevention theory of Fishbein and Ajzen (1975) with the social reinforcement and learning theory of Bandura (1977), the social norms/problem behavior theory of Jessor and Jessor (1977), and the developmental theory of Rosenberg (1979).

Interventions based on the traditional rational teaching model had a significantly greater effect on knowledge than did the other models. However, other interventions had greater positive impact on attitudes and tobacco and alcohol behavior than the rational model. Bruvold and Rundall suggest that a threshold change in knowledge is necessary for behavior change, but attitude changes (in the desired direction) do not necessarily follow from knowledge changes. A combination of new knowledge and attitude changes is more certain to produce behavioral results. Traditional didactic approaches are less effective than other means—social reinforcement, normative, or developmental approaches—in generating the sequence of attitudinal and behavioral changes. Bruvold and Rundall concluded (1988: 72-73): "If an individual receives peer praise and support for refusing cigarettes, the individual will become fully convinced that such refusals lead to peer praise and support, a desirable outcome . . . ." Interventions targeted at self-esteem enhancement, if they appropriately followed the tenets of this theory, would be directed at providing the individual more constant and explicit feedback from significant other peers.

A meta-analysis by Hansen et al. (1990) was based on 85 distinct cohorts of subjects. The results reveal that sample retention decreases over time: the mean proportion of subjects retained in the analyses decreased from 81.3 percent to 67.5 percent from follow-ups taken at 3 months and 3 years, respectively. There was considerable variability in the rates of attrition between studies. The greatest drop in sample retention was found to occur during the first year of investigation. The authors concluded that researchers should interpret their results in light of the rate of attrition and should further their efforts to reduce the rate of attrition. The results of Project ALERT, discussed later in this chapter, are particularly subject to this conclusion.

Summary

Tobler's, Bangert-Drowns's, and Bruvold and Rundall's results converge on the general ineffectiveness of knowledge-only, affective-only, and knowledge-plus-affective programs in affecting alcohol or drug use behaviors. Hansen et al. (1990) provide a warning on long-term effects due to the attrition of subjects over time. Tobler and Bangert-Drowns diverge on what kind of trainers seem best to induce informational or attitudinal change, but these results may simply reflect the different kinds of programs analyzed. Tobler's review suggests that programs oriented toward peer relationships gain in efficacy, but it leaves open the question of what this advantage consists of and whether it actually applies to drug prevention programs among general student populations. The strength of Tobler's meta-analysis is its overview of different program types, but the strongest conclusion is difficult to regard as applicable to prevention programs at all. These results suggest that we need to examine studies of prevention interventions that employ much more tightly defined contents and more careful scientific designs than appear typical among the types of studies that carry so much weight in some of the meta-analyses. A good set of cases in point for preferred studies are the Life Skills Training Program, several studies using a cognitive-behavioral approach, and the Napa Drug Abuse Prevention Project. In each case, the research involved programs with discrete modular characteristics, applied to full grade cohorts, within closely controlled experimental protocols.

THREE PROGRAMS MEETING TOBLER'S CRITERIA

Life Skills Training Program

Life Skills Training (LST) is a middle-school curriculum with three components (Botvin and Wills, 1985; Botvin and Eng, 1982; Botvin et al., 1983):

- Substance-specific information and refusal skills training;

• A personal skills component to improve critical thinking and responsible decision making, help cope with anxiety, and learn principles of self-improvement; and

• Improvement of nonverbal and verbal communication skills for social encounters including dating, conversation, and assertiveness.

The Life Skills Training program was implemented with booster sessions among a predominantly white sample of 7th grade students who were followed up in grades 8 and 9 (Botvin et al., 1990). Using a randomized block design, schools were assigned to receive one of three programs: (1) the LST program with formal provider training and implementation feedback, (2) LST with videotaped provider training and no feedback, or (3) no treatment. Program outcomes showed significant reduction in smoking and marijuana use in both experimental conditions at the first and second year follow-up. The program did not have significant effects on drinking frequency or amount, although at second year follow-up there was a significant effect on the frequency of getting drunk for the experimental groups who received videotape teacher training. The effect was strongest for cigarette use; this is not surprising, as the intervention was originally designed for smoking prevention. These findings provide the most rigorous test of the LST approach and demonstrate the effectiveness of LST in reducing substance-using behaviors among youth in grades 7 to 9.

There is further evidence of short-term efficacy of the LST approach to drug prevention. The program reduced the proportion of smoking among a sample of black urban youths by 56 percent in a 3-month posttest (Botvin et al., 1989a). A skills training program for smoking prevention was tested in a predominantly Hispanic population; preliminary evidence supported the efficacy of the program (Botvin et al., 1989b). These findings suggest that a preventive approach with some short-term effectiveness in white middle-class populations may be generalizable to minority populations.

There is some evidence of long-term efficacy using the LST approach with regard to cigarettes. Smoking prevention integrated into a primary cancer center prevention strategy with diet modification revealed that the rate of initiation of cigarette smoking was significantly lower in treatment schools 6 years following the intervention (Walter et al., 1989). In grade 4 no smokers were present in the intervention and nonintervention groups; the rate of initiation of cigarette smoking was 73.3 percent less (3.5 versus 13.1 percent) among youths in the intervention schools than those in nonintervention schools; and the effect was stronger for males than for females. An 8-year follow-up study in Finland (North Karelia Youth Project) revealed that the positive short-term effects on smoking prevalence found immediately following the intervention and in a 4-year follow-up diminished by the 8-year follow-up. The difference in smoking prevalence, however, remained significant for the community-wide and direct program schools in comparison to control schools (Vartiainen et al., 1990). The effect was stronger for the community-wide program than for the direct program approach implemented in schools without community-wide activities. Almost one-half of youth in control schools (47 percent) smoked, compared with 37 percent of those in the direct program schools and 31 percent in the community-wide program schools.

In summary, the research findings support short- and long-term efficacy of Life Skills Training with respect to knowledge, attitudes, and cigarette smoking outcomes of youth in different ethnic populations and in schools and community settings.

The Cognitive-Behavioral Approach

Positive effects on knowledge, attitudes, and behavior have been reported for the cognitive-behavioral approach to drug prevention. In a study of 5th and 6th graders (N = 741), the self-control skills group reported less weekly cigarette smoking and revealed better scores on measures of communication, self-instruction, self-praise, cigarette refusals, and noncompliance to smoke cigarettes at the 15-month follow-up (Gilchrest et al., 1986). Similar results were found in a smaller study (N = 65) of 6th graders in two middle schools. The average number of cigarettes smoked per week was lower at posttest, 6-month, 12-month, and 24-month follow-ups (Schinke et al., 1986). This approach has been found effective in populations of Native American youths with posttest and 6-month follow-up results showing positive outcomes on measures of substance use knowledge, attitudes, and self-reported rates of tobacco, alcohol and drug use (Schinke et al., 1988). Similarly, Native American youths receiving the intervention revealed better knowledge scores on drug effects and interpersonal skills for managing pressure to use drugs and reported lower rates of alcohol, marijuana, and inhalant use (Gilchrist et al., 1987).

The cognitive-behavioral approach to drug abuse prevention has focused exclusively on school-based programming. Compared with the social influences and life skills approaches, the efficacy of the cognitive-behavioral approach has been established on relatively small sample sizes. The long-term efficacy of the cognitive-behavioral approach has not been established, nor has its full potential been exploited. The approach has recently been applied to the prevention of HIV infection among African American and Hispanic youths (Schinke et al., 1990).

The Napa Drug Abuse Prevention Project

The Napa project, implemented in Napa County, California, was designed to evaluate the effectiveness of seven school-based substance abuse prevention strategies. Four of the strategies were in-service teacher training courses that focused on classroom and individual factors thought to influence attitudes toward school, self-esteem, and the development of social competencies. None of these four courses addressed the topic of drug use per se. The in-service teacher training strategies were designed to improve the classroom management skills of teachers and to provide a more positive and socially rewarding learning environment within the classroom; these achievements, in turn, would presumably affect drug-oriented attitudes and behaviors. The four strategies included:

Magic Circle, in which teachers were trained to lead structured small-group discussions on particular topics designed to improve students' communications skills and their understanding of themselves and others (grades 3-4).

Effective Classroom Management/Elementary, in which teachers were taught various communication skills, discipline techniques, and self-concept enhancement techniques (grades 4-6).

Effective Classroom Management/Junior High, in which communication, discipline, and self-concept enhancement skills were adapted for teaching in the junior high environment (grades 7-9).

Jigsaw, in which teachers were taught to organize classrooms into co-operative learning groups of five or six students in which each student teaches an essential piece of the regular curriculum to the other group members (grades 4-6).

Two alternative strategies were offered as elective academic courses to junior high school students. In these courses, students were taught certain skills and provided opportunities for helping peers or younger children. These courses, too, did not address the topic of drug use; instead, they sought to strengthen self-concepts and to teach social competencies.

Cross-Age Tutoring, in which students tutored younger children on a regular basis in reading and other academic subjects (grades 8-9).

Operating a School Store, in which students ran a school store on campus selling school supplies and snacks, while learning relevant business skills in a related academic course (grades 8-9).

The final strategy was a course in *Drug Education*. This course taught social competencies and drug information to 7th graders. In the final version of the 12-session (45 minutes per session) course, taught by a health educator, students learned Maslow's (1980) framework for understanding motivation, learned a systematic decision-making process, analyzed techniques used in commercial advertising, learned assertiveness skills for dealing with peer pressure, and practiced setting personal goals. Toward the end of the course, students were also provided information about tobacco, alcohol, and marijuana in response to their written questions. Students applied social skills in considering drug use issues. It should be noted that the *Drug Education* curriculum incorporates virtually all of the elements identified as important to the social influence approach (e.g., the Project ALERT lessons; see Chapter 2 and below), although in a somewhat different sequence.

One or more separate evaluations of each strategy were conducted during the course of the Napa project, covering variables of classroom and school environment, personal satisfaction among students, perceived peer norms and behavior, and specific drug attitudes, beliefs, knowledge, and behavior. In some studies, two or three strategies were applied to the same group of students over 2- or 3-year periods. Schaps and colleagues (1984), the evaluators, found that none of the six nondrug-specific strategies evaluated in the Napa project produced a pattern of positive outcomes. There were no effects on attitudes or perceptions of self, peers, classroom climate, or the school experience; no effects on attendance or academic achievement; no significant changes in perceptions of peer group norms or drug-related attitudes or behaviors. The *Drug Education* curriculum showed some short-term positive effects on 7th grade girls in one of two studies (but not on 8th-grade girls), and no positive results for boys in either grade. The one set of positive effects was no longer discernible at the 1-year follow-up.

Schaps and associates concluded that these prevention strategies were ineffective because some were inadequately or inconsistently implemented and others were based on inadequate theories of prevention. For example, process evaluation showed that *Effective Classroom Management* skills were infrequently used by teachers, apparently because these skills were incompatible with routine teaching practices and styles. In even the most "exemplary" *Jigsaw* classrooms, there were no effects on students compared with controls, nor were any effects observed in fully operationalized *Cross-Age Tutoring* or *School Store* programs. The Napa results were further confirmed in a meticulous study by Hansen and colleagues (1988), who conducted a 2-year trial with experimental and control groups comparing an affective education curriculum with a social influences curriculum. They too found that affective intervention was clearly less effective. In fact, students receiving the affective education intervention had even higher rates of substance use at follow-up than those in the control group. A plausible explanation for these findings was that none of the affective-type interventions was based on a clear vision or model of the specific pathways to drug use—the predisposing, enabling, and reinforcing elements. Mild nondrug-specific curriculum augmentation on a few grade levels simply may not reach deeply enough into the lives of children, especially those most at risk, to change the likely trajectories of their behavior. Instead of viewing this as ruling out the school as a site for intervention, some have looked to evidence from more comprehensive efforts at school modification; we return to this line of research later in the chapter.

DO LARGE-SCALE SOCIAL INFLUENCE PROGRAMS WORK?

The results of the meta-analyses by Tobler and Bangert-Drowns, reinforced by the Napa project and the work of Hansen and colleagues, suggest that modular, nondrug-specific affective programs are not effective. They leave open the possibility that modular programs recognizably conforming to the social influence approach may be effective. A series of large-scale programs—that is, programs applying to cohorts of large sample sizes—have appeared in recent years. It is instructive to give detailed attention to two of these programs that have sustained high methodological standards, one focusing strictly on cigarette smoking prevention, the other on all of the gateway drugs: the Waterloo study in east-central Canada and Project ALERT in the western United States.

Waterloo

In two school districts in Waterloo, Ontario, 22 schools volunteered to participate in a study of an antismoking intervention using social influence. Eleven were assigned, mostly at random, to the experimental condition; the others served as controls. The study students were in grades 6-8 and provided questionnaire and saliva samples at pretest, immediate posttest, and at end of the 6th, beginning and end of the 7th, and end of the 8th grades. Total attrition plus absenteeism was less than 10 percent per year; 67 percent of students provided data at all six data points (Flay, 1985; Flay et al., 1989).

Pretest differences between the two groups were minimal, and no group differences were observed for baseline smoking behavior. The program was found to have its major effect on those students in the experimental schools who were judged at high initial risk because they had parents, siblings, or friends who smoked. For example, among high-risk students who had never tried smoking prior to pretest, by the end of 8th grade, 67 percent of those in the program group versus 22 percent of controls still had never smoked, 6 percent of the program group versus 39 percent of controls were experimental smokers, and none of the program students versus 6 percent of controls were regular smokers (Best et al., 1984). Program effects varied over time. The greatest immediate effects were on those already experienced with smoking, but there were later effects on those with no or little smoking experience at pretest.

In a 6-year follow up, 90 percent of the subjects were tracked in the

11th and 12th grades, and 80 percent provided data (Flay et al., 1989). Significant program effects that had been observed earlier (including follow-ups only one or two grades earlier) had decayed into statistical insignificance by the latter high school years. Whether the dependent variable is smoking at all or smoking heavily at follow-up, program effects were no longer significant. The best predictors of smoking status at the 6-year follow-up were: (1) pretest smoking behavior and (2) the pretest level of social risk (as defined above) for becoming a smoker.

Flay and colleagues (1989:1374) conceded: "The lack of significant preventive effects by grade 12 raises the question of the value of the social influences approach for smoking prevention." (High school follow-up data from a very similar study in Minnesota closely parallel the results observed in Waterloo—Murray et al., 1989.) The researchers caution, however, against an interpretation of the latest findings as evidence that prevention efforts have no effect on results 6 years later, when the proper conclusion should be that results obtained early had disappeared 6 years later in the absence of sustained or repeated efforts. The decay of effects over a 6-year period might not be ineluctable; this process might be counteracted by modest intermediary efforts; for example, brief booster sessions in the early high school years may be sufficient to perpetuate the substantial early effects; this would be in line with advances over the 10 years since the Waterloo study was initiated with respect to understanding essential components of effective prevention programs. Such enhancements warrant at least the working hypothesis that more current versions of social influence programming could produce more durable effects, a hypothesis in line with Bangert-Drowns's finding that more recent techniques seem to produce greater effects. In addition, broader social norms and policies have grown more supportive of nonsmoking; students in the control schools may have been endogenously exposed to many elements of the social influence approach in recent years, thus catching up with their experimental peers and obscuring the effects of the older program. Finally, even if smoking rates had equalized at a point in time 6 years later, the delayed onset of smoking in the treated cohort could have a valuable delayed effect, namely, a greater tendency to quit smoking in early and middle adulthood.

Project ALERT

Project ALERT was an $8 million study funded by the Conrad N. Hilton Foundation and conducted by a research team at RAND Corporation. It tested the effects of an education program focused explicitly on resistance to cigarettes, alcohol, and marijuana, using a carefully designed and executed experimental procedure to evaluate the effects of the curriculum. The researchers recruited 30 junior high and middle schools in eight cooperating school districts in Oregon and California, which spanned urban, suburban, and rural locations and included large variations in ethnic and socioeconomic characteristics.

The researchers administered questionnaires with a variety of baseline test items and collected saliva to test for nicotine metabolite in the entire cohort of 7th grade students in the 30 schools, generating a baseline group of 6,527 students. Each school was randomly assigned (with some restrictions to ensure balanced samples) to one of three conditions. In 10 of the experimental schools, health educators taught the 8-session ALERT curriculum to the 7th grade classes and the following year delivered three booster sessions in 8th grade. In another 10 schools, trained "teen leaders" assisted the health educators in delivering these lessons. In the remaining 10 schools there was no intervention, although previously instituted information-type drug prevention programs continued during the study period in four of these schools.

The research group monitored implementation to be certain the experimental sessions took place and all lesson elements were delivered (actually 92 percent were delivered in monitored sessions). The researchers administered follow-up retest items concerning alcohol, marijuana, and cigarette use at 3, 9, and 15 months after baseline, the last follow-up coming after the booster sessions were completed. About 59 percent of the baseline sample completed all three retests and were included in the analysis of outcomes— a rather disappointing follow-up rate for such a meticulously conceived study.

Logistic regression was used to control for baseline differences among students and schools and isolate the treatment effect of the two experimental approaches. Based on earlier research, particularly the results of Chassin (1984) and Botvin, Resnick, and Baker (1983), the authors (Ellickson et al., 1988; Ellickson and Bell, 1990) hypothesized that:

- The program would affect cigarette and marijuana smoking more than alcohol use;
- Teen leaders would improve the effectiveness of the curriculum;
- Booster sessions would enhance or better preserve program effects; and
- The program would be more effective for students who were nonusers or "experimenters" than those reporting regular use.

The latter hypothesis about differential effects according to subgroup, although opposite to the Waterloo findings, was held so powerfully that all of the outcome analyses were divided to report effects on three levels of risk groups per baseline drug use. For cigarettes and alcohol, respectively, the risk groups were defined as follows:

- Current users (past-month),
- Ever-users (but only once or twice, and not currently), and
- Never-users;

In the case of marijuana, the baseline risk groups were as follows:

- Marijuana ever-users,
- Marijuana never/cigarette ever-users, and
- Marijuana never/cigarette never-users.

The authors abstract the results of the study in the following rather positive light, albeit with a caveat (Ellickson et al., 1988:vii-viii; cf. Ellickson and Bell, 1990):

> Project ALERT effectively prevented or reduced cigarette and marijuana use among young adolescents in our sample. The rate of marijuana initiation in the Project ALERT schools was one-third lower than that in the control schools. Regular and daily smoking by students who had not experimented with cigarettes before being exposed to the program were reduced by as much as 50 to 60 percent. These effects were reinforced or enhanced by the booster sessions offered in eighth grade. The program was equally effective in schools with substantial minority populations and in predominantly white schools.
>
> However, Project ALERT is by no means a panacea that would eliminate adolescent drug use. While it was initially successful against alcohol, the early gains in alcohol prevention had eroded by the time students reached eighth grade. Also, it was not effective with previously confirmed cigarette smokers, who actually smoked more after being involved in the program. This boomerang effect, however, was strictly limited to cigarette smoking.

These very carefully phrased results focus on particular subgroups and particular individual transitions. Curiously, there is no report of the overall effect of the curriculum, taking all subgroups together; that is, it is unclear how the cohort as a whole responded, even though the treatments were delivered en bloc to students in all subgroups, and the authors do not propose a mechanism for presorting students according to the analytically defined risk groups.

These findings reinforce a concern about results reported by Botvin and associates (1982, 1983, 1989a) for their Life Skills Training curriculum for junior high school or high school sophomore students: although data were generally collected for students who had initiated smoking prior to receiving the intervention, these groups are systematically excluded from Botvin and colleagues' analyses.

The published data are not complete enough to reconstruct fully the main (whole-group) effects of Project ALERT, but they do permit a fairly good approximation of overall outcomes in each of the three conditions for each drug. When these estimated main effects are taken into account, a more conservative statement of the findings seems appropriate. In the untreated control schools, at the final test point in grade 8, current use of alcohol, cigarettes, and marijuana (at least once in the past month) was reported by 48 percent, 22 percent, and 13 percent, respectively, of 8th grade students. In the experimental schools, at the same point in time— after completion of the 2-year curriculum—the comparable figures for the adult-taught and adult/teen-taught schools were 46 and 48 percent for alcohol, 22 and 23 percent for cigarettes, and 10 and 11 percent for marijuana.

Reports of relatively intensive alcohol, cigarette, and marijuana use yielded similar patterns but at lower percentages of the 8th grade classes: the control versus experimental group comparisons are 5.8 versus 5.6/6.3 percent (weekly alcohol), 2.9 versus 3.3/4.0 percent (daily cigarettes), and 2.0 versus 1.8/1.4 percent (weekly marijuana). The implied cell sizes for weekly marijuana are in the 20-30 range, and the p of this and other differences is certainly above .10. All of these 8th-grade consumption rates, and the 7th grade baselines, are well above national and regional norms derived from retrospective reports by high school seniors.

It appears, then, that the ALERT curriculum had virtually no net effect either on alcohol use (the effect was consistently lacking across all baseline subgroups) or on cigarette smoking (here the positive and negative effects in two of the three subgroups cancelled each other out, and there was no net effect in the third subgroup, comprising half the students). The net effect of the curriculum on marijuana use—a reduction in the neighborhood of one-sixth to one-fourth—is large enough to draw attention (the probability of avoiding a type I error is almost certainly acceptable, because cell sizes reach 110 and 140). But methodological considerations warrant particular caution concerning the effects of the curriculum on marijuana use in this study. The overall sample attrition was 41 percent from baseline, and the attrition of baseline marijuana ever-users was the highest for any preintervention characteristic—61 percent missing at follow-up. In this light, a 2-3 percent difference in posttest marijuana use among those remaining in the sample cannot be considered definitive.

Despite the positive indications yielded by earlier studies and the strong theoretical underpinnings of social influence programs, two of the largest trials, representing best practice at the time they were designed, conducted by excellent research teams, have yielded results that must be viewed as discouraging. While these trials, inaugurated some years ago, do not necessarily represent the most advanced work that might be fielded today, they give a good indication of the degree to which school-based prevention programming is operating on the basis of plausibility and good faith rather than research knowledge. To make these points even more emphatically, it is worthwhile to examine the state of knowledge concerning the effectiveness of the two most widely disseminated school-based programs today: *DARE* (Drug Abuse Resistance Education), a social-influence program, and *Here's Looking at You*, a series of curriculum packages originally based on affective education, which now incorporates most of the social influence model as well.

DARE

The 17-week DARE curriculum was developed in 1984 as a joint effort between the Los Angeles Police Department and the Los Angeles Unified School District. It is based to a large extent on the SMART curriculum (see Hansen et al., 1988) and thus resembles the social influence curriculum being delivered as STAR in Kansas City and I-STAR in Indianapolis (see Pentz et al., 1989b) (described in a later section). The DARE program is delivered primarily to 5th or 6th graders, although there are K-3 as well as junior high/middle school components. At the present time, DARE is offered in over 450 cities throughout the United States and in several other countries; in some states the program is statewide.

Several unique aspects of the DARE program should be noted. The curriculum is taught by uniformed police officers instead of teachers. Officers receive an intensive, 80-hour, structured training course covering the curriculum contents and associated teaching techniques. Officers are taught in all their training to "go by the book," and this instruction, along with the paramilitary character of police training in general, provides a greater probability of strict fidelity to the curriculum. (Process evaluations by Clayton et al., 1991, on one site revealed strong fidelity to the curriculum and excellent classroom skills among police officers delivering the curriculum.) Implementation of the DARE program requires a working relationship between the school system and the police department in a community, an arrangement that has potential benefits for the community at large.

Published evaluations of the DARE program are scarce at this point in time. DeJong (1987) evaluated the program with 7th grade students in Los Angeles. His findings suggest that DARE students accepted significantly fewer offers to use drugs and reported significantly lower levels of substance use than nonequivalent control group students. DeJong's study was an after-only design and there was no random assignment into treatment and control conditions.

An evaluation of the DARE program in North Carolina (Ringwalt et al., 1990) focused on pre-posttest differences for students attending 10 randomly selected DARE schools and 10 randomly selected control schools. The DARE program had no significant effect on self-reported drug use, intentions to use drugs, or self-esteem. Significant differences in the appro-

priate direction did appear in attitudes toward drug use in general and toward specific drugs, in perceptions of peers' attitudes toward drug use, in
assertiveness, and in recognizing media influences to use drugs.

Faine and Bohlander (1988) examined pre-posttest differences between
DARE and non-DARE students controlling for type of school (rural, paro-
chial, inner-city, and suburban). Self-reported use of drugs was not examined. Self-esteem and attitudes toward the police were significantly different between all DARE and all non-DARE students. However, when controls
for types of school were instituted, the differences were not uniformly significant. There were significant differences between treatment and control
students in perceived external control, which remained when statistical controls for type of school were implemented. The DARE curriculum did have
the desired effect of producing significantly greater scores on peer resistance skills.

An evaluation of DARE conducted among 400 inner-city youth in Nashville
(Faine, 1989) found no support for the effectiveness of the DARE curriculum in changing peer resistance or positive attitudes toward drugs. In this
study, DARE students had significantly more negative attitudes toward the
police than the non-DARE students at posttest.

Clayton and associates (1991) are engaged in a five-year, cohort sequential study of the effectiveness of DARE in Lexington, Kentucky. In the
first cohort, 23 schools were randomly assigned to receive the DARE curriculum; 8 schools were randomly assigned to the control condition (i.e.,
students received the standard health curriculum, which contained a drug
education unit). In the remaining cohorts, all students received the DARE
curriculum. A difficulty from a diffusion standpoint (see Best et al., 1988)
is that, once a school system makes a commitment to implement a prevention intervention, it is virtually impossible to convince them to allow for
control schools. In a pre-posttest analysis, Clayton et al. (1991) found
statistically significant effects on general attitudes toward drugs, negative
attitudes toward specific drugs (e.g., cigarettes, alcohol, marijuana), and on
a scale measuring peer relationships. Expected differences in self-esteem
and peer pressure resistance were not observed, although for the latter the
results were close to the conventional criterion of statistical significance.
There were no statistically significant differences in self-reported drug use,
although this may have been affected by low base rates, a problem endemic
to this type of research.

Here's Looking at You

The original version of the Here's Looking at You program was designed to help young people find responsible ways of dealing with alcohol
in their environment by relying on decision-making skills. The curriculum

was aimed at enhancing knowledge about alcohol, self-esteem, coping, and decision making (Hochheimer, 1981; Hawkins et al., 1986).

Here's Looking at You Two is a modification of the original curriculum and was integrated into a variety of different subjects (versus health classes only). Its objectives were expanded toward helping adolescents (grades 9-12) make responsible decisions regarding the use of alcohol and drugs. The curriculum, consisting of 20 lessons, attempts to help students gain basic information about alcohol and drugs, to be able to express their feelings, and to understand their values and behavior in relation to alcohol and other drugs. This particular intervention was adopted in schools throughout the United States.

The current version, Here's Looking at You 2000, was introduced in 1986. This intervention is composed of 150 lessons to be spread out over grades K-12. The goals are to provide information on substances, to develop social skills, and to encourage bonding to school, family, and community. The component on drug information is focused on the gateway drugs (tobacco, alcohol, and marijuana). Building social skills is focused on making friends and staying out of trouble and alerts students to the risk of having drug-using friends (Rogers et al., 1989).

The initially encouraging evaluation of Here's Looking at You by Mauss and colleagues (1981) included experimental and control schools and covered 3 years. The most positive results occurred for students first exposed to the curriculum in grade 6 who continued to receive it through grade 8. Enhanced self-esteem, knowledge about alcohol, and decision-making skills were sustained across the duration of the study. A persistent impact was reported for problem drinking (that is, adverse consequences precipitated by drinking episodes), although not for the quantity and frequency of drinking. A notable finding was that peers, parents, and religiosity had a stronger predictive power over outcome variables than exposure to the curriculum.

The evaluators noted that students receiving the curriculum appeared to "lose ground less rapidly to peer influence" than those who were in the control schools. This was expected to influence rates of experimental use of drugs. On the basis of the evaluation, Mauss et al. (1981) recommended that prevention interventions should occur prior to middle school, before the establishment of drinking-related attitudes and behavior, and that greater emphasis should be laid on intervention components focused on peers and parents (see Hawkins et al., 1986).

The Here's Looking at You curriculum was reexamined by Hopkins et al. (1988) over 3 years in a sample of 6,808 students in grades 4-12 from five school districts in the Northwest. Data were collected at pretest, posttest, and annual follow-up periods from students attending experimental and control schools. No statistically significant impact on measured outcomes was noted either in the short term or long term. Hopkins et al. (1988) concluded that this curriculum is not effective in preventing alcohol use or abuse.

Swisher and his colleagues (1985) evaluated Here's Looking at You Two among predominantly white, middle-class 8th graders in experimental and control schools in Pennsylvania. The two schools had a total of 869 students and were similar in distribution on gender and other characteristics. Use of tobacco, marijuana, and stimulants was significantly lower in the school receiving the prevention intervention. The differences approached statistical significance for use of liquor and depressants. There were lower rates of drinking to become drunk and or "high" in the experimental school. The actual frequency of drinking was not lower among students in the experimental school, but the reported amount used per occasion was lower.

Subsequently, the Here's Looking at You Two curriculum was evaluated by Green and Kelly (1989) among 1,698 experimental and 1,005 control students in elementary, middle, and high school grades in five school districts. Pretest, posttest, and follow-up data indicate a significant increase in knowledge about alcohol and drugs at the elementary and middle levels, but less effect on underlying attitudes about use and use itself. Few significant differences emerged with regard to key targets of this curriculum (e.g., self-esteem, decision making, coping skills). The authors suggest lack of fidelity in implementation as a possible explanation.

In summary, research results on Here's Looking at You are inconsistent. The only replicated result is a more "responsible" use of alcohol among treated students—they don't drink less, but they appear to drink in ways that are less damaging to themselves. The contradictory results in other respects are not explained, and the great expansion of the size and scope of the program package and its widespread diffusion to schools around the country seems entirely out of proportion to the evidence of its usefulness in preventing drug problems.

RESEARCH IN PROGRESS

Developmental Interventions

The developmental approach to intervention outlined in Chapter 2 involves deep-seated shifts in the organization of the school, designed to produce far more than simple reductions in drug incidence and prevalence. This intervention is part of a larger movement of school reform. Higher overall educational achievement is part of its goal structure, but more as an expected consequence of prosocial achievement than as an end in itself. Two outstanding research programs employ interventions approaching the theoretically indicated degree of comprehensiveness: the Seattle Social Development Project and the Child Development Project in Northern California. Each of these programs involves substantial training of teachers and a parent program.

The Seattle Social Development Project is a longitudinal field experiment in an economically and ethnically diverse population of public school students (Hawkins and Catalano, 1987). The theoretical model underlying the program hinges on social bonding. The program is designed to promote bonding with school and family by recognizing and rewarding prosocial behavior, increasing communication and positive interaction with adults and other children at home and in school, and improving school performance. The program teaches parents how to promote children's academic and social development and helps teachers establish a classroom environment more conducive to learning and self-control. Practices such as interactive teaching and cooperative learning are intended to increase opportunities for all students to succeed academically.

Students and teachers in 12 elementary and middle schools were assigned randomly to treatment and control conditions in 1981 and have been followed longitudinally since then. Fifth grade students compared with controls had more positive attitudes toward school, more positive attachments to family members and teachers, and more discussion of problems at home with parents. Seventh grade students had higher academic achievement, fewer suspensions and expulsions, and less self-reported use of drugs at school.

The Child Development Project is a comprehensive elementary curriculum implemented in a suburban middle-class school district in 1982 and a heterogeneous urban district in 1988. The program includes classroom, schoolwide, and family components designed to promote prosocial behavior by building a caring community within the school, making the curricula more accessible and engaging, and building family bonds. Major classroom elements include a literature-based reading program that highlights core values and interpersonal understanding, a cooperative learning strategy that aims to build internalized motivation and satisfaction, and a disciplinary approach that emphasizes relationship-building, rational explanation, and mutual problem-solving rather than contingent rewards and punishments.

The suburban program has been extensively evaluated. Observational data in classrooms show the expected program effects on spontaneous prosocial behavior (Solomon et al., 1988) and capability to resolve hypothetical conflicts (Battistich et al., 1989); lower loneliness and anxiety, higher peer acceptance, and more democratic beliefs; and higher reading comprehension in tests of higher-order thinking skills. The program has not been in effect long enough for statistically sufficient levels of drug behaviors to emerge so that differences between treatment and control schools can be assessed.

Midwestern Prevention Project

This particular project, initiated in 1984 in Kansas City and known as Project STAR, is being replicated in Indianapolis as I-STAR. The data published to date are from Kansas City. The overall design in Kansas City is a 6-year study. Pentz and associates (1989a) describe the components as resistance skills training and environmental support of nonsmoking and nondrug use through the use of school, parent, and community organization programs, health policy changes, and mass media programming. To date, however, the only program components in effect (or reported on) are "a 10 session youth educational program on skills training for resistance of drug use, 10 homework sessions involving active interviews and role-plays with parents and family members, and mass media coverage" (Pentz et al., 1989b: 3260). During a 16-month program period, a total of 16 television, 10 radio, and 30 print media events for the project were broadcast over the metropolitan area.

The sampling design was complicated. The subjects consisted of the entire 6th and 7th grade cohort in 16 schools, and 25 percent of the cohort, sampled randomly by classrooms, in 34 schools. However, "seventy percent of the sample was tracked by grade cohort (cross-sectional sampling of available students in the cohort, including new incoming students who might not have received the intervention; average n = 3371); the remaining 30% was tracked by individual (n = 1607)" (Pentz et al., 1989b:3262).

In 1985 and 1986, 6 of the 50 schools were no longer active in the study and 2 schools missed data collection because of scheduling conflicts. This left 42 schools in the reported final sample. Of these, 8 had been assigned randomly to either program or control conditions, 20 had agreed to reschedule existing programming and were assigned to receive the intervention, and 14 were either unable or unwilling to reschedule existing programming and thus were designated as control schools (along with the 4 randomly assigned to the control condition). In the control schools, the classroom intervention was delayed by a year, and thus was delivered to the cohorts *after* those sampled by the researchers.

Using as a base the 1,607 students who constituted the individuals specifically tracked, Pentz et al. (1989b:3262) estimated that 3.1 percent had provided no follow-up at any time after baseline and 84 percent were assessed at both baseline and 1-year follow-up. In a report using data from all 42 schools, Pentz et al. (1989b) reported prevalence rates for use of cigarettes, alcohol, and marijuana that were significantly lower at 1-year follow-up in the intervention condition relative to the delayed intervention condition. This held true regardless of whether controls were implemented for race, grade, socioeconomic status, or urbanicity. The effects were 17 versus 24 percent for cigarette use, 11 versus 16 percent for alcohol use in the past month, and 7 versus 10 percent for marijuana use in the past month. The net increase in prevalence of drug use in the intervention schools was one-half the net increase observed in the delayed-intervention (control) schools.

Using complete data from 1,244 subjects from the STAR project in Kansas City, Dwyer et al. (1989) reported 8 versus 18 percent in the 1-year follow-up prevalence rates for past-week cigarette smoking, mixed evidence of an effect on marijuana use, and no evidence of an effect on alcohol use. At 2 years, 12 percent of treatment versus 19 percent of control students reported smoking in the week preceding the data collection. There were also program effects across different levels of cigarette use ranging from no current use to use of one pack or more per day at the 2-year follow-up.

Further 3-year follow-up findings reveal that the prevention programs were effective in reducing tobacco and marijuana use and in reducing the prevalence of drug use in youth identified at high and low risk (Johnson et al., 1990). The authors conclude that a comprehensive community-based approach to drug abuse prevention is effective in preventing the onset of substance abuse, the benefits of which are accrued by high- and low-risk populations.

Five-year follow-up results from Kansas City were released in June 1990; 24 percent of the treated students reported smoking cigarettes in the preceding month compared with 32 percent of the control students. Some 36 percent of students who received the STAR curriculum reported having used alcohol in the preceding month compared with 50 percent of the control students. The results regarding past month use of marijuana were 14 percent for those students who had received STAR compared with 20 percent who had received the curriculum taught to control students. In separate analyses from eight schools in which students were tracked over time, 1.6 percent of the treatment students compared with 3.7 percent of the control students reported past month use of cocaine, including crack.

The Midwestern Prevention Project is one of the most ambitious drug abuse intervention efforts undertaken to date. It aims to utilize a whole-community approach, and it targets different institutional spheres of influence (e.g., schools, family, media, community institutions) for a consistent message. Unlike many prior and contemporary efforts at drug abuse prevention interventions, results from the Midwestern Prevention Project in Kansas City indicate solid, statistically significant effects on all three gateway drugs: cigarettes, alcohol, and marijuana. These effects seem to have persisted for up to 5 years following the intervention. These are the most unequivocal results produced by any social influences (or any other kind of) prevention program to date. However, the multifaceted nature and complexity of the project has created a number of potential methodological confounds and concerns.

Most generally, the sampling and selection process was neither random nor clearly described. While the investigators have attempted to address questions about sampling by pointing to evidence of initial equivalence of experimental and control groups, the tests for initial equivalence reported to date have been limited to several demographic characteristics and baseline rates of reported use. It is possible that sampling bias is obscured by presentation of data for individuals and that what is crucial for assessing concerns about sampling are data at the school level.

Furthermore, concerns exist about implementation. The investigators indicate reasonably strong fidelity to the curriculum, but the process data reported to date are sparse, more often based on assertion than measurement. The investigators report on the number of media events that occurred with regard to the Midwestern Prevention Project. However, no data on actual exposure to the media events nor evidence of attention and response to these messages has been presented. The investigators also report an exceedingly high estimate of parental involvement in the homework assignments that are an integral part of the curriculum, but have not indicated how these data were obtained or their validity or reliability checked.

Summary

The major work in progress reported here on developmental programs and the most recent large-scale study of a social influence curriculum have not yet progressed to the point of changing the generally restrained position of earlier research regarding the effectiveness of known school-based prevention methods. The recent shift in research focus from within-classroom interventions to broader school reforms is consistent with the growing recognition of the need to support educational interventions on the drug problem with broader policy and environmental changes and to engage parents, community, and other social forces.

MASS MEDIA AND DRUG ABUSE PREVENTION

Rogers and Storey (1987:818-821) indicate that ". . . a minimal definition of a communication campaign would have to include four characteristic features: (1) a campaign is purposive; (2) a campaign is aimed at a large audience; (3) a campaign has a more or less specifically defined time limit; and (4) a campaign involves an organized set of communication activities." By this definition, the sporadic efforts through the mass media since 1954 to reduce smoking have been a series of campaigns rather than a cohesive campaign. They have been impressive in their correspondence to the peaks and troughs in the more than 40 percent decline in adult male smoking since the first surgeon general's report on smoking and health (U.S. Department of Health, Education and Welfare, 1964).

Each drug abuse prevention campaign essentially attempts to inform individuals in the audiences about drugs, persuade them about the dangers and consequences of use or abuse, and to mobilize overt behavioral change (e.g., never to start or to quit). But like the smoking campaigns, they must be viewed in the larger historical context of various media activity as well as news events and program initiatives at all levels of national, state, and local organization.

A number of objectives attach to any communications campaign. Various models have been developed to describe the intermediate variables and to explain how the objectives are achieved. In the context of marketing new products, Ray (1973) described a cognitive, affective, conative hierarchy of communication effects. McGuire's (1968) model includes the concepts of attention, comprehension, yielding, retention, and action. Fishbein and Ajzen's (1975) model includes belief, attitude, intention, and behavior. Rogers (1983) describes the decision process about innovation in terms of knowledge, persuasion, decision, and confirmation stages.

There have been several eras in views about communications campaigns. The first era involved a somewhat naive view of the monolithic influence of the media. As Rogers and Storey (1987:831) indicate: "In the early eras of communication campaigns there was frequent reliance on mass media alone to accomplish campaign objectives. The shifting conceptualization of communication effects and of the communication process had led to recognition that communication operates within a complex social, political, and economic matrix, and that communication could not be expected to generate effects all by itself."

The more recent recognition that communication campaigns and media effects are embedded within a broad and varied range of other stimuli and forces has moved this field beyond simple typologies. Roberts and Maccoby (1985:543) note: "Recognition of the multidimensionality of media effects has led to more complex conceptualization of effects, including not only consideration of their nature (e.g., cognitions, attitudes, behaviors), but also such dimensions as time, unit of analysis, degree of content specificity (e.g., a specific behavior versus a class of behaviors), and type of impact (e.g., establishing, changing, or stabilizing a response). Finally, there is a growing theoretical attention to identification and elaboration of the role of third variables in the media-effects relationship."

Research has been conducted on at least two levels of media effects. One of these is broad in scope and has generally been targeted at the national level seeking evidence of change in awareness, knowledge, attitudes, behavioral intention, and behavior. A second level at which research has been conducted is at the development and implementation level, which is generally more basic and formative in nature.

In a 1983 report, Flay and Sobel reviewed the state of the art regarding the role of mass media in preventing adolescent drug abuse. They conclude (1983:17): "An overwhelming majority of mass media drug abuse prevention programs have failed to change behavior. One obvious reason for this is that most [public service announcements] campaigns literally fail to even reach the audience. . . . Another reason for the failure of most PSA campaigns has probably been heavy reliance on information and fear messages. . . . Another problem with anti-drug-abuse campaigns was the tendency for PSAs to be directed to unidentifiable audience segments."

Flay and Sobel (1983:18-22) identify three macro-level mediators of success and failure in drug abuse prevention campaigns. They are whether program dissemination occurs at propitious times, selectivity or individual predispositions to attend to the message, and whether the message is boosted with interpersonal communications regarding the issue or problem of concern.

Flay et al. (1983) evaluated a smoking prevention program targeted at junior high school students and their families. It was a multifaceted program that involved five 5-minute segments on the early evening news hour, a 5-day classroom curriculum with an emphasis on skills for resisting social influences, home and family activities coordinated with the school-based and media intervention, followed by a series of five 5-minute segments on smoking cessation. They found greater effects on program than control students with regard to knowledge, attitudes, behavioral intention, and actual reported smoking behavior.

Flay (1987) reviewed evaluations of 40 mass media programs or campaigns designed to influence cigarette smoking. Programs and campaigns that were informational and motivational in nature did affect awareness, knowledge, and attitudes. Extensive national campaigns providing information on consequences of smoking and encouraging attempts to quit have had measurable effects on smoking prevalence and quitting rates. For example, Warner (1989) claims that, in the absence of antismoking campaigns, adult per capita consumption of cigarettes in 1987 would have been an estimated 79 to 89 percent higher than the levels actually measured. Flay (1987) reports mixed results from programs and campaigns designed to promote specific behavioral attempts to quit smoking.

In the drug abuse field, there has been a concerted effort to ensure the priority of drug abuse on the public policy agenda via the "Just Say No" campaigns and the focus on cocaine and the cocaine hotline of the National Institute on Drug Abuse. These campaigns seem to have had the desired impact in terms of exposure and coverage as well as behavioral responses measured by hotline calls (see Forman and Lachter, 1989; Shoemaker et al., 1989).

Currently, the Partnership for a Drug-Free America is conducting a major antidrug campaign. The stated goal is to help "unsell" illegal drug use in the United States. Two strengths of this campaign are the voluntary involvement and commitment of the advertising industry in developing the messages and the extensive formative research that has provided a foundation for the messages and the campaign.

The evaluation of effectiveness of these campaigns involves matched samples of persons interviewed annually for three consecutive years (1987, 1988, 1989). It should be noted that these are not longitudinal samples; different persons were interviewed each year. The samples (children ages 9-12, teenagers ages 13-17, and adults) were recruited in malls or central locations via a technique known as the mall intercept method. The college students were interviewed in central campus locations on 130 college campuses. There is an attempt to weight the samples with census data on age. In addition, there is a partitioning of the data into high-media-exposure and low-media-exposure areas determined by the extent of media exposure of Partnership messages.

None of the methods or data have yet been peer-reviewed. However, Black (1989) has reported that there are positive and statistically significant impacts on both attitudes and self-reported behavior overall, and that "teenagers appear to be the most resistant to advertising messages in general, although changes have shown marked improvement over the three years of the study. It is harder to link this effect to the advertising in 1989 than it was in 1988." There are observed differences in the predicted direction with regard to effects on knowledge, attitudes, and behavior in the high-media versus the low-media areas.

Although it has received a great deal of public and media attention, there are significant limitations in the evaluations of the Partnership for a Drug-Free America campaign. First, the data are generally gathered from persons who are intercepted in shopping malls and other central gathering places. In spite of the fact that the evaluators attempt to adjust the sample to census data, adjustment is made only for age. This is simply not an adequate sampling methodology for testing the effectiveness and impact of such a campaign. With regard to college students, there are representatives from 130 campuses. However, again the data were collected from convenience samples of students found in common areas.

Second, in comparing self-reported drug use among mall intercept samples in high-media with those in low-media areas, there is a leap in inference from media exposure (a universalistic and macro-level measure) to self-reported drug use (an individual-level measure). This is an example of what has been called the ecological fallacy, attributing changes in individual behavior obtained from independent samples to a macro-level change or variable. Third, the data are presented in only a descriptive and, for the most part, univariate format. More sophisticated statistical analyses would allow for a more realistic appraisal of the impact of the messages on attitudes and behavior.

Donohew et al. (1990b:25) provide a succinct summary of the practical difficulties involved in achieving behavioral change using television spots. "Anti-drug PSAs, which have become an increasingly popular tool in prevention campaigns, are submerged in an often overwhelming clutter of programming and product advertisements and must be capable of: (1) immediately attracting the attention of target audience members; and (2) motivating these viewers to attend to the remainder of the message. In addition, such messages require relatively high levels of information processing intensity and/or involvement to achieve informational and persuasive goals. Adding to these problems, motives for watching television ordinarily do not include exposure to advertising or PSAs."

Donohew et al. (1990a) started their research program with a laboratory setting and the measurement of psychophysiological responses to certain kinds of media messages. The key variables in their research have been sensation seeking and the sensation value of the message. The assumption behind their research has been that people high on sensation seeking are at greater risk for drug use than low sensation seekers. On this premise, prevention messages should help move the more vulnerable group toward recreations, lifestyles, and occupations that compete more effectively with drugs in satiating these needs. Although amusement parks, active sports or exercise participation, and highly mobile or nonroutinized jobs are not surefire antidotes or immunizations against drugs, research on sensation seeking argues for the potential value of these types of alternatives.

Donohew et al. (1990a:22) indicate that: "If the goal of the media campaign is modest behavioral change, such as inducing young adults to call a hotline for drug-related information or to put them in touch with face-to-face intervention programs, then this study offers clear guidelines for designing messages to reach nondrug users with different needs for sensation. For high sensation seeking non-users, a group whose members are particularly at risk to become users, a message which stresses exciting alternatives to drug use and is high in sensation value clearly is more likely to be effective than one which stresses peer resistance skills and is lower in sensation value. . . . Low sensation seeking non-users, on the other hand, appear to be much more influenced by a message which stresses peer resistance skills and is low in sensation value than by a message which features exciting alternatives to drug use and is high in sensation value."

A major strength of this project is that formative evaluation is an integral part of the process. The fact that this study began in the laboratory and used reasonably large samples as well as physiological responses to messages provides a solid foundation for subsequent expansions of effort. In addition, identification of sensation seeking as the primary characteristic to be used in targeting messages is unique in that most efforts at audience segmentation have focused on sociodemographic factors.

However, there are some potential limitations that should be mentioned. First, this project relies heavily on sensation seeking as the most important predictor of drug use. Donohew and his colleagues found a relatively strong and general relationship between sensation seeking and use of various drugs. However, there are questions in the existing literature about this relationship. For example, Huba et al. (1981) found that the several dimensions of sensation seeking are differentially related to use of different drugs. Therefore, the relationship may be specific according to drug, not a general one between the sensation seeking construct and all drug use. In another analysis, Newcomb and Bentler (1988) examined the relationship of alcohol use and delinquency, controlling for the underlying personality factor of sensation seeking. The hypothesis was that the alcohol-delinquency relationship would be spurious because of the influence of sensation seeking. This was not the case. Second, the practice by Donohew et al. (1990a) of grouping subjects into high and low sensation-seeking categories on the basis of a median split ignores the alleged multidimensionality of the construct. This characteristic of a potential audience also will make it difficult to pinpoint a population for purposes of audience segmentation. Third, the use of messages that are either high on sensation value or low on sensation value, while related to drug use propensity in the laboratory, may be less differentiating in the real world amidst all the clutter that accompanies the delivery of the message as well as the context within which the message is received. Fourth, the data are either sparse to nonexistent regarding the relationship of sensation seeking to something other than initiation of drug use (e.g., continuation, maintenance, progression within classes of drugs, progression across classes of drugs, regression, cessation, and relapse).

All research efforts have limitations, however; the research by Donohew and his colleagues constitutes a viable model for the process of linking messages to targeted audiences. This is an important concept. Roberts and Maccoby (1985:542) describe this orientation: "Current thinking also views the power of the media as highly conditional, depending on a variety of contingent and/or contributory third variables. Chaffee (1977) discusses a trend away from research concerned with demonstrating effects on only 10 percent of a full population toward studies suggesting a 100 percent effect on a specifiable group that may comprise only 10 percent of the population. In other words, recent models posit powerful media effects limited by specifiable (and empirically demonstrable) conditions." The goal then should be a closer linkage of the formative process of developing messages with existing research on the etiology of drug use and abuse.

Rogers and Storey (1987:836-840) have identified nine features of effective mass media campaigns against drug abuse:

• *Widespread exposure* to campaign messages is a necessary ingredient in a communication campaign's effectiveness.

- The mass media can play an important role in *creating awareness-knowledge*, in *stimulating interpersonal communication*, and in *recruiting* individuals to participate in campaign activities.
- Interpersonal communication through *peer networks* is very important in leading to and maintaining behavior changes.
- The *perceived credibility* of a communication source or channel enhances the effectiveness of a communication campaign.
- *Formative evaluation* can improve the effectiveness of campaigns by producing messages that are specific to the desired behavior change.
- *Campaign appeals* that are socially distant from the audience member are not effective.
- *Campaigns promoting prevention* are less likely to be successful than those with immediate positive consequences.
- *Audience segmentation strategies* can improve campaign effectiveness by targeting specific messages to particular audiences. Audience segmentation strategies have focused almost entirely on sociodemographic characteristics or on specific drugs such as cocaine. The next step will be to use the existing literature on risk and protective factors to identify individuals at higher risk for drug use or abuse and target messages specifically at these groups. In fact, this is the basis for the Donohew et al. (1990a) emphasis on high sensation seeking, an identified risk factor for drug use.
- *Timeliness and accessibility* of media and interpersonal messages can contribute to campaign success.

These characteristics of effective messages provide an important beginning point for future research on media effects on drug use and abuse and in antidrug prevention campaigns. However, the guiding principle of the entire enterprise has been identified by Roberts and Maccoby (1985:544): ". . . the ubiquity and assumed homogeneity of media content can make one forget that meanings are not in messages, but in people."

There are at least three lessons that have been learned from prior research. First, media alone are much less effective than media messages employed in the context of a broad campaign that includes the use of interpersonal channels. Second, there is a need for targeting or audience segmentation. Third, there is a strong need for formative research in message and campaign design.

The media are only one tool in the hands of those concerned with drug abuse prevention, albeit a very important one.

CONCLUSIONS AND RESEARCH NEEDS

The only way to determine if something really works is to try it, in a way that permits objective evaluation. Systematic testing and evaluation are essential to progress in reducing drug abuse. A clear majority of the research published as evaluations of the effectiveness of preventive interventions is methodologically weak. Corrections of their weaknesses is not a matter of applying rigid formulae. It requires patient commitment to attracting quality researchers to the field; applying stringent requirements to publications and research grants, and urging other research sponsors, collaborators (such as school administrators), reviewers, and publication editors to attend to them; developing and supporting appropriate research training; and attending to socioenvironmental aspects and data quality control elements of proposed research.

Social Influence Research

Much of the work on social influence approaches to interventions completed to date has focused on preventing or delaying onset of use of the gateway drugs. But preventing or delaying onset is only part of the drug using and abusing continuum. The entire continuum of transitions in drug use (e.g., initiation, continuation, progression, regression, cessation, relapse) constitute the proper focus of attention for prevention interventions (Clayton, 1992).

A number of major methodological issues need to be addressed directly and critically. The first of these is attrition. While attrition rates are often reported, the analyses usually show demographic and pretest differences on gross drug use measures between those who remained in the studies and those who dropped out of the study by treatment condition. Very few researchers examine or report such differences on the major predictive or mediating variables. The attrition rates in longitudinal studies on prevention fall below rates achieved by large-scale national studies such as High School and Beyond, Monitoring the Future, and the National Education Longitudinal Study. It is essential that panel studies meet attrition standards that amount to the state of the art in survey research.

A second major methodological issue is statistical power. Most evaluations of prevention interventions suffer from a lack of statistical power to detect differences. When significant main effects fail to emerge, it is common to make too much of subgroup differences. A third major methodological issue concerns contamination. In the United States, it is virtually impossible to find a true no-treatment control group. However, none of the studies describes the prevention intervention received by the so-called control group members.

Clayton and Cattarello (1990) have identified a series of implementation issues concerning social influence curricula that should receive attention. Standards for reporting implementation information scarcely exist, and too often it is virtually impossible to say what actually occurred in an intervention (Moskowitz, 1989). A set of standards such as those discussed by Clayton and Catalano should be promulgated as an evaluation criterion for NIDA-sponsored intervention research.

It is clear that different curricula are being used by different researchers, but explicit comparisons are just beginning to be made (see Rogers et al., 1989). Comparing the efficacy of different social influence programs, for example, may be comparing the proverbial apples and oranges until standard descriptive frameworks and measures of what actually occurs in the classroom are developed, tested, and widely used. There may be different pedagogical strategies employed even by teachers or trainers working from the same book in adjacent classrooms delivering, presumably, the same lessons. These differences may be systematically related to the different roles occupied by those delivering the curriculum; to date the evidence on role effects (peer leaders, health educators, classroom teachers, counselors or mental health professionals, substance abuse specialists, police officers) is a raft of inconsistencies. A methodological initiative is needed to develop a gauge of trainers' ability to communicate content accurately, intelligibly, and in ways consistent with the theory intended to be applied by the intervention.

The skills being taught in these interventions require different levels of ability for abstraction and specificity. There is little research on how a single curriculum teaching such skills affects youth in a grade cohort who have attained different developmental levels. There are few instances in which research projects have measured actual individual student exposure to the prevention intervention, to see whether exposure level is connected to measured outcomes; if there is an individual dose-response effect, this would substantially raise our confidence that outcomes and program features were indeed causally linked. It is also important to find some way to assess the degree to which curriculum is embedded in the school milieu.

Finally, we add our concern to that of Kozlowski et al. (1989:455) and Flay (1985) about advocacy for social influence interventions in the absence of even moderately compelling evidence of efficacy.

Ethnicity and Gender: The Neglected Dimensions

Most school-oriented drug prevention programs are based on mainstream, one-size-fits-all cultural assumptions. Data on differential effects by ethnicity of recipient students have been notably scarce in evaluations of major school-based prevention programs; either no disaggregation by ethnicity is provided by the evaluators, or the sample sizes for which data are available are too small for any differential zero-order or partially controlled effects to be statistically discernible. Differentiation of effects by gender is more common, and there are glimmers of evidence that prevention programs are more effective with girls. One might assume that girls are a population that is more compliant to begin with, but assumptions will not take the place of deeper investigation.

An important exception to the rule of not reporting ethnic results is Graham and colleagues (1990), who evaluated short-term program effects of a social influence program (SMART) among Los Angeles 7th graders. There was a significant program effect for Asian students, nonsignificant positive effects for Hispanic and black students, and null effects for white students. There were group differences with respect to different drugs. Moreover, virtually all positive program effects were among girls, suggesting that gender role norms interact strongly with ethnic group differences.

Koepke et al. (1990) found that in a cigarette smoking prevention and cessation program addressed to middle school students and their parents in San Diego and Los Angeles counties (where one-fifth of all Hispanics in the United States reside), black parents and children were more likely than white, Hispanic, or Asian ones to assess the parents as potentially effective in preventing their children from smoking, but Hispanic parents were more likely to implement "say no" teaching.

School-based drug prevention programs that are not based on one-size-fits-all models but rather on culturally specific tailoring do exist, and these have been described to some extent in the literature. Most are adjunctive to a community-based program; however, none has been satisfactorily evaluated to date using well-designed outcome measures to test their effectiveness (Orlandi, 1986). There have been some evaluations among community-based prevention programs; for example, Schinke and colleagues (1988) pilot-tested a program of culturally specific training in competence skills using random-assignment designs among bicultural Native Americans living on reservations; they reported desired effects on drug use prevalence. We will return to issues of cultural and community specificity in the appendix, where we provide a more elaborate discussion of how research can be structured to yield more usefully articulated results taking these specificities into account.

Generic Interventions

Substance abuse is nested within a range of other high-risk activities, and it is highly plausible that progress in reducing the most serious levels of illicit drug use will require broad rather than narrow interventions. There is evidence throughout the prevention literature that training in resistance skills and information on health risks may be relatively puny if not counterproductive forces in the lives of many high-risk children, compared with other problems that may overwhelm them. In studies relevant to substance abuse, intensive interdisciplinary programs that deal with more central aspects of their behavior show promise to meaningfully improve the prospects of these young people, although the specific effects on drug problems are as yet unknown.

REFERENCES

Bandura, A.
1977   *Social Learning Theory.* Englewood Cliffs, N.J.: Prentice Hall.
Bangert-Drowns, R.L.
1988   Effects of school-based substance abuse education: a meta analysis. *Journal of Drug Education* 18(3):243-264.
Battistich, V., D. Solomon, M. Watson, J. Solomon, and E. Schaps
1989   Effects of an elementary school program to enhance prosocial behavior on children's cognitive social problem-solving skills and strategies. *Journal of Applied Developmental Psychology* 10:147-169.
Bell, C.S., and R. Battjes
1987   *Prevention Research: Deterring Drug Abuse Among Children and Adolescents.* NIDA Research Monograph 63. Rockville, Md.: National Institute on Drug Abuse.
Best, J.A., B.R. Flay, S.M.J. Towson, K.B. Ryan, C.L. Perry, K.S. Brown, M.W. Kersell and J.R. d'Avernas
1984   Smoking prevention and the concept of risk. *Journal of Applied Social Psychology* 14(3):257-273.
Best, J.A., S.J. Thomson, S.M. Santi, E.A. Smith, and E.S. Brown
1988   Preventing cigarette smoking among school children. *Annual Review of Public Health* 9:161-201.
Black, G.S.
1989   The Attitudinal Basis of Drug Abuse. The Third Year. Report prepared for the Partnership for a Drug Free America. Gordon S. Black Corporation, Rochester, New York.
Botvin, G.J., and A. Eng
1982   The efficacy of a multicomponent approach to the prevention of cigarette smoking. *Preventive Medicine* 11:199-211.
Botvin, G.J., and T.A. Wills
1985   Personal and social skills training: cognitive-behavioral approaches to substance abuse prevention. Pp. 8-49 in C.S. Ball and R. Battjes, eds., *Prevention Research: Deterring Drug Abuse Among Children and Adolescents.* NIDA Research Monograph 63. Rockville, Md.: National Institute on Drug Abuse.
Botvin, G.J., N.L. Resnick, and E. Baker
1983   The effects of scheduling format and booster sessions on a broad spectrum psychosocial approach to smoking prevention. *Journal of Behavioral Medicine* 6(4):359-379.
Botvin, G.J., H.W. Batson, S. Witts-Vitale, V. Bess, E. Baker, and L. Dusenbury
1989a   A psychosocial approach to smoking prevention for urban black youth. *Public Health Reports* 12(3):279-296.
Botvin, G.J., L. Dusenbury, S. James-Oritz, and J. Kerner
1989b   A skills training approach to smoking prevention among Hispanic youth. *Journal of Behavioral Medicine* 12(3):279-296.
Botvin, G.J., E. Baker, L. Dusenbury, S. Tortu, and E.M. Botvin
1990   Preventing adolescent drug abuse through a multi-modal cognitive-behavioral approach: results of a 3-year study. *Journal of Consulting and Clinical Psychology* 58(4):437-446.
Bruvold, W.H., and T.G. Rundall
1988   A meta analysis and theoretical review of school based tobacco and alcohol intervention programs. *Psychology and Health* 2:53-78.

Chaffee, S.H.
1977   Mass media effects: new research perspectives. Pp. 210-241 in D. Lerner and L. Nelson, eds., *Communication Research—A Half Century Appraisal.* Honolulu: East-West Center Press.

Chambers, J., and E. Morehouse
1983   A cooperative model for preventing drug and alcohol abuse. *National Association of Secondary School Principals Bulletin* 81-87.

Chassin, L.
1984   Chapter in P. Karoly and J. Steffen, eds., *Adolescent Behavior Disorders.* Lexington, Mass.: Lexington Books.

Clayton, R.R.
1992   Transitions in drug use: risk and protective factors. Pp. 15-51 in M. Glanz and R. Pickins, eds., *Vulnerability to Drug Abuse.* Washington, D.C.: American Psychological Association.

Clayton, R.R., and A. Cattarello
1990   Prevention intervention research: the challenges and opportunities. In C. Leukefeld and W. Bukoski, eds., *Drug Abuse Prevention Intervention Research: Methodological Issues.* Rockville, Md.: National Institute on Drug Abuse.

Clayton, R.R., A. Cattarello, L.E. Day, and K.P. Walden
1991   Persuasive communications and drug prevention: an evaluation of the D.A.R.E. program. In H. Sypher, L. Donohew, and W. Bukoski, eds., *Persuasive Communication and Drug Abuse Prevention.* Boston: Erlbaum.

DeJong, W.
1987   A short-term evaluation of project DARE (Drug Abuse Resistance Education): preliminary indications of effectiveness. *Journal of Drug Education* 17(4):279-294.

Donohew, L., E. Lorch, and P. Palmgreen
1990a   Sensation seeking and targeting of televised anti-drug PSAs. In L. Donohew et al., eds., *Persuasive Communication and Drug Abuse Prevention.* Hillsdale, N.J.: Lawrence Erlbaum and Associates.

Donohew, L., P. Palmgreen, E. Lorch, and W.F. Skinner
1990b   Personal communication.

Dwyer, J.H., D.P. MacKinnon, M.A. Pentz, B.R. Flay, W.B. Hansen, E.Y.I. Wang, and C.A. Johnson
1989   Estimating intervention effects on longitudinally observed health behaviors: the Midwestern Prevention Project. *American Journal of Epidemiology* 130:781-795.

Ellickson, P.L., and R.M. Bell
1990   Drug prevention in junior high: a multi-site longitudinal test. *Science* 247:1299-1305.

Ellickson, P.L., R.M. Bell, M.A. Thomas, A.E. Robyn, and G.L. Zellman
1988   *Designing and Implementing Project ALERT: A Smoking and Drug Prevention Experience.* Santa Monica, Calif.: Rand Corporation.

Faine, J.R.
1989   D.A.R.E. in Nashville Schools. Western Kentucky University Social Research Laboratory, Bowling Green, Kentucky.

Faine, J.R., and E. Bohlander
1988   Drug Abuse Resistance Education: An Assessment of the 1987-88 Kentucky State Police DARE Program. Western Kentucky University Social Research Laboratory, Bowling Green, Kentucky.

Fishbein, M., and I. Ajzen
1975   *Belief, Attitude, Intention, and Behavior: An Introduction to Theory and Research.* Reading, Mass.: Addison-Wesley.

Flay, B.R.
  1985   What we know about the social influences approach to smoking prevention: re-
        view and recommendations. Pp. 67-112 in C.S. Bell and R. Battjes, eds., *Preven-
        tion Research: Deterring Drug Abuse Among Children and Adolescents.* NIDA
        Research Monograph No. 63. Rockville, Md.: National Institute on Drug Abuse.

Flay, B.R.
  1987   Mass media and smoking cessation: a critical review. *American Journal of Public
        Health* 77(February):153-160.

Flay, B.R., and J.L. Sobel
  1983   The role of mass media in preventing adolescent substance abuse. Pp. 5-35 in T.J.
        Glynn et al., eds., *Preventing Adolescent Drug Abuse: Intervention Strategies.*
        NIDA Research Monograph 47. Rockville, Md.: National Institute on Drug Abuse.

Flay, B.R., C.A. Johnson, W.B. Hansen, L.M. Grossman, J.L. Sobel, and L.M. Collins
  1983   Evaluation of a School-Based, Family-Oriented, Television-Enhanced Smoking
        Prevention and Cessation Program: The Importance of Implementation Evalua-
        tion. Paper presented at the joint meeting of Evaluation Network and the Evalua-
        tion Research Society, Chicago.

Flay, B.R., K. Koepe, S.J. Thomson, S. Santi, A. Best, and S.K. Brown
  1989   Six year followup of the first Waterloo school smoking prevention trial. *American
        Journal of Public Health* 79(10):1371-1376.

Forman, A., and S.B. Lachter
  1989   The National Institute on Drug Abuse cocaine prevention campaign. Pp. 13-20 in
        P.J. Shoemaker, ed., *Communication Campaigns About Drugs: Government, Me-
        dia, and the Public.* Hillsdale, N.J.: Lawrence Erlbaum Associates.

Gilchrist, L.D., S.P. Schinke, J.K. Bobo, and W.H. Snow
  1986   Self-control skills for preventing smoking. *Addictive Behaviors* 11:169-174.

Gilchrist, L.D., S.P. Schinke, J.E. Trimble, and G.T. Cvetkovich
  1987   Skills enhancement to prevent substance abuse among American Indian adoles-
        cents. *International Journal of the Addictions* 22:869-879.

Glass, G., B. McGaw, and M. Smith
  1981   *Meta-Analysis in Social Research.* Beverly Hills, Calif.: Sage Publications.

Goplerud, E., ed.
  1991   *A Practical Guide to Substance Abuse Prevention in Adolescence.* OSAP Preven-
        tion Monograph 8. DHHS Pub. No. (ADM)91-1725. Washington, D.C.: U.S.
        Government Printing Office.

Graham, J.W., C.A. Johnson, W.B. Hansen, B.R. Flay, and M. Gee
  1990   Drug use prevention programs, gender and ethnicity: evaluation of three seventh-
        grade Project SMART cohorts. *Preventive Medicine* 19(3):305-313.

Green, J.J., and J.M. Kelly
  1989   Evaluating the effectiveness of a school drug and alcohol prevention curriculum:
        a new look at "Here's Looking at You Two." *Journal of Drug Education* 19(2):117-
        132.

Hansen, W.B., C.A. Johnson, B.R. Flay, D. Phil, J.W. Graham, and J. Sobel
  1988   Affective and social influences approaches to the prevention of multiple substance
        abuse among seventh graders: results from Project SMART. *Preventive Medicine*
        17(2):135-154.

Hansen, W.B., N.S. Tobler, and J.W. Graham
  1990   Attrition in substance abuse prevention research. *Evaluation Review* 14(6):677-
        685.

Hawkins, J.D., and R.F. Catalano
  1987   The Seattle Social Development Project: Progress Report on a Longitudinal Pre-

vention Study. Paper presented at the National Institute on Drug Abuse Science Press Seminar, Washington, D.C.

Hawkins, J.D., D.M. Lishner, and R.F. Catalano, Jr.
1986   Childhood predictors and the prevention of adolescent substance abuse. Pp. 75-125 in C.L. Jones and R.J. Battjes, eds., *Etiology of Drug Abuse: Implications for Prevention.* NIDA Research Monograph No. 56. Rockville, Md.: National Institute on Drug Abuse.

Hochheimer, J.L.
1981   Reducing alcohol abuse: a critical review of education strategies. Pp. 286-335 in M.H. Moore and D.R. Gerstein, eds., *Alcohol and Public Policy: Beyond the Shadow of Prohibition.* Washington, D.C.: National Academy Press.

Hopkins, R.H., A.L. Mauss, K.A. Kearney, and R.A. Weisheit
1988   Comprehensive evaluation of a model alcohol education curriculum. *Journal of Studies on Alcohol* 49(1):38-50.

Horan, J.J., and J.M. Williams
1982   Longitudinal study of assertion training as a drug abuse prevention strategy. *American Educational Research Journal* 19(3):341-351.

Huba, G.J., J.A. Wingard, and P.M. Bentler
1981   A comparison of two latent causal variable models for adolescent drug use. *Journal of Personality and Social Psychology* 40:180-193.

Jessor, R., and S.L. Jessor
1977   *Problem Behavior and Psychosocial Development: A Longitudinal Study of Youth.* New York: Academic Press.

Johnson, C.A., M.A. Pentz, M.D. Weber, J.H. Dwyer, N. Baer, D.P. MacKinnon, W.B. Hansen, and B.R. Flay
1990   Relative effectiveness of comprehensive community programming for drug abuse prevention with high-risk and low-risk adolescents. *Journal of Consulting and Clinical Psychology* 58(4):447-457.

Koepke, B.L., B.R. Flay, and C.A. Johnson
1990   Health behavior and minority families: the case of cigarette smoking. *Family Community Health* 13(1):35-43.

Kozlowski, L.T., R.B. Coambs, R.G. Ferrence, and E.M. Adlaf
1989   Preventing smoking and other drug use: let the buyer beware and the interventions be apt. *Canadian Journal of Public Health* 80:452-456.

Kumpfer, K.L.
1987   Special populations: etiology and prevention of vulnerability to chemical dependency in children of substance abusers. Pp. 1-73 in B. Brown and A. Mills, eds., *Youth at High Risk of Substance Abuse.* DHHS Pub. No. (ADM)87-1537. Rockville, Md.: National Institute on Drug Abuse.

Maslow, A.
1980   *Motivation and Personality.* New York: Harper and Row.

Mauss, A.L., R.H. Hopkins, R.A. Weisheit, and K.A. Kearney
1981   *A Longitudinal Evaluation of the "Here's Looking at You" Alcohol Education Program.* Final Report. Social Research Co., Pullman, Washington.

McGuire, W.J.
1968   Personality and susceptibility to social influence. Pp. 1130-1187 in E.F. Borgatta and W.W. Lambert, eds., *Handbook of Personality Theory and Research.* Chicago: Rand McNally.

Moskowitz, J.M.
1989   Guidelines for reporting outcome evaluation studies of HPDP programs. In M.T. Braverman, ed., *Evaluating Health Promotion Programs.* San Francisco: Jossey Bass.

Murray, D.M., P. Pirie, R.V. Luepker, and U. Pallonen
  1989   Five- and six-year follow-up results from four seventh-grade smoking prevention
          strategies. *Journal of Behavioral Medicine* 12:207-218.
Newcomb, M.D., and P.M. Bentler
  1988   *Consequences of Adolescent Drug Use.* Beverly Hills, Calif.: Sage Publications.
Orlandi, M.A.
  1986   Community-based substance abuse prevention: a multicultural perspective. *Jour-
          nal of School Health* 56()9):394-401.
Pentz, M.A., D.P. MacKinnon, B.R. Flay, W.B. Hansen, C.A. Johnson, and J.H. Dwyer
  1989a   Primary prevention of chronic diseases in adolescence: effects of the Midwestern
          Prevention Project on tobacco use. *American Journal of Epidemiology* 130:713-
          724.
Pentz, M.A., J.H. Dwyer, D.P. MacKinnon, B.R. Flay, W.B. Hansen, E.Y.I. Wang, and C.A.
          Johnson
  1989b   A multicommunity trial for primary prevention of adolescent drug abuse. *Journal
          of the American Medical Association* 261:3259-3266.
Ray, M.
  1973   Marketing communication and the hierarchy of effects. Pp. 147-176 in P. Clarke,
          ed., *New Models for Communication Research.* Beverly Hills, Calif.: Sage Publi-
          cations.
Ringwalt, C., S. Ennett, and K. Holt
  1990   An outcome evaluation of Project D.A.R.E. Personal correspondence, March. 1.
Roberts, D., and N. Maccoby
  1985   Effects of mass communication. Pp. 539-598 in G. Lindzey and E. Aronson, eds.,
          Handbook of Social Psychology, Vol. 2: Special Fields and Applications. New
          York: Random House.
Rogers, E.
  1983   *Diffusion of Innovations*, 3rd ed. New York: Free Press.
Rogers, E.M., and J.D. Storey
  1987   Communication campaigns. Pp. 817-846 in C.R. Berger and S.H. Chaffee, eds.,
          Handbook of Communication Science. Beverly Hills, Calif.: Sage Publications.
Rogers, T., B. Howard-Pitney, and B.L. Bruce
  1989   *What Works? A Guide to School-Based Alcohol and Drug Abuse Prevention
          Curricula.* Health Promotion Research Center. Palo Alto, Calif.: Stanford Center
          for Research in Disease Prevention.
Rosenberg, M.
  1979   *Conceiving the Self.* New York: Basic Books.
Schaps, E., J. Moskowitz, J. Malvin, and G. Schaffer
  1984   *The Napa Drug Abuse Prevention Project: Research Findings.* DHHS Publica-
          tion No. ADM(84)1339. Rockville, Md.: National Institute on Drug Abuse.
Schinke, S.P., L.D. Gilchrist, R.F. Schilling, W.H. Snow, and J.K. Bobo
  1986   Skills methods to prevent smoking. *Health Education Quarterly* 13(1):23-28.
Schinke, S.P., G.J. Botvin, J.E. Trimble, M.A. Orlandi, L.D. Gilchrist, and V.S. Locklear
  1988   Preventing substance use among American-Indian adolescents: a bicultural com-
          petence skills approach. *Journal of Counseling Psychology* 35:87-90.
Schinke, S.P., A.N. Gordon, and R.E. Weston
  1990   Self-instruction to prevent HIV infection among African-American and Hispanic-
          American adolescents. *Journal of Consulting and Clinical Psychology* 58(4):432-
          436.
Shoemaker, P.J., W. Wanta, and D. Leggett
  1989   Drug coverage and public opinion, 1972-1986. Pp. 67-80 in P.J. Shoemaker, ed.,

Communication Campaigns About Drugs: Government, Media, and the Public.
Hillsdale, N.J.: Lawrence Erlbaum Associates.

Solomon, D., M.S. Watson, K.E. Delucchi, E. Schaps, and V. Battistich
1988 Enhancing children's prosocial behavior in the classroom. *American Educational Research Journal* 25:527-554.

Sorensen, J., and S. Jaffe
1975 An outreach program in drug education: teaching a rational approach to drug use. *Journal of Drug Education* 5(2):87-96.

Swisher, J.D., C. Nesselroade, and C. Tatanish
1985 Here's Looking at You Two is looking good: an experimental analysis. *Humanistic Education and Development* (Mar):111-119.

Tobler, N.S.
1986 Meta analysis of 143 adolescent drug prevention programs: quantitative outcome results of program participants compared to a control or comparison group. *Journal of Drug Issues* 16(4):537-567.

Tobler, N.S.
1989 Drug Prevention Programs Can Work: Research Findings. Unpublished manuscript, School of Social Welfare, State University of New York, Albany.

U.S. Department of Health, Education and Welfare
1964 *Report of the Advisory Committee to the Surgeon General on Smoking and Health.* Public Health Service. Washington, D.C.: U.S. Department of Health, Education and Welfare.

Vartiainen, E., U. Fallonen, A.L. McAlister, and P. Puska
1990 Eight-year follow-up results of an adolescent smoking prevention program: the North Karelia Project. *American Journal of Public Health* 80(1):78-79.

Wachter, K.W., and M.L. Straf, eds.
1990 *The Future of Meta-Analysis.* New York: Russell Sage Foundation.

Walter, H.J., R.D. Vaughan, and E.L. Wynder
1989 Primary prevention of cancer among children: changes in cigarette smoking and diet after six years of intervention. *Journal of the National Cancer Institute* 81(13):995-999.

Warner, K.
1989 Effects of an anti-smoking campaign: an update. *American Journal of Public Health* 79(February):144-151.

Wunderlich, R., J. Lozes, and J. Lewis
1974 Recidivism rates of group therapy participants and other adolescents processed by a juvenile court. *Psychotherapy: Theory, Research and Practice* 2(3):243-245.

Appendix

Community Settings and Channels for Prevention

Practitioners and researchers in a variety of fields, from agricultural extension to public health, have come to think that prevention planners and practitioners should work from a series of fundamental propositions: (1) Begin from a base of community ownership of the problems and the solutions; (2) plan thoroughly using relevant theory, data, and local experience as bases for program decisions; (3) know what types of interventions are most acceptable and feasible to implement (in the absence of certainty about what is most effective) for specific populations and circumstances; (4) have an organizational and advocacy plan to orchestrate multiple intervention strategies into a complementary, cohesive program; and (5) obtain feedback and evaluation of progress as the program proceeds (Abrams et al., 1986; Bracht, 1990; Breckon et al., 1989; Dignan and Carr, 1986; Green and Kreuter, 1991).

These general propositions have had sufficient testing in a number of areas to be called "principles of practice" (Bracht and Kingsbury, 1990). Whether they have sufficient research support to be considered theoretical propositions, however, is debated by experienced practitioners and research scientists (Glanz et al., 1990; Thompson and Kinne, 1990). The first principle, for example, would qualify as a corollary of the theory of participation. That is, cumulative research in educational psychology and various applied fields demonstrates with some consistency that cognitive, affective, and behavioral changes in learners or clients are greater in response to interventions when the subjects engage actively rather than passively, agree on the purpose of the change (especially when convinced that the purpose serves their own goals, relates to their own values, and meets their own perceived needs), control the pace and content of the intervention, monitor results, and obtain direct and immediate feedback on their own performance. These highly generalizable tenets of the theory of participation apply in classroom, worksite, recreational, and clinical settings as well as in community-wide interventions (Bracht and Kingsbury, 1990; Green, 1986; Hunt, 1990; Minkler, 1990).

The relevance and application of these broad generalizations to drug abuse prevention bear further study. The principles tend to be applied, sometimes intuitively, by drug abuse prevention planners and practitioners, but their analysis by researchers has been unsystematic (Holder and Giesbrecht, 1989; Room, 1989). Drug abuse prevention research could learn from and contribute much to the evolving body of prevention research on health and human services. This appendix examines the prevention literature on a variety of health and human service fields related to drug abuse. Our purpose is to draw implications whenever possible between other bodies of prevention research and the prospects for drug abuse prevention through various community-based channels and settings. Promising community-wide interventions are examined first, followed by specific settings within communities including schools, families, work sites, and medical care settings. We seek, in particular, to identify gaps in knowledge that could be most fruitfully addressed by drug abuse prevention research.

COMMUNITY INTERVENTIONS

We distinguish here between community interventions and interventions in communities. The differences are two: (1) the comparative magnitude and scope of the undertaking, as determined by the size and diversity of the group or population for whom the program is intended and (2) the number of organizations and levels of organization involved.

Defining Community

The term *community* has various meanings. In the context of professional practice or research, it is necessary to choose an explicit, operational definition. In this discussion, community is defined in structural and functional terms. Structurally, a community is an area with geographic and often political boundaries that are demarcated as a county, a metropolitan area, a city, a township, a neighborhood, or a block (Holder and Giesbrecht, 1989). Functionally, a community is a place where "members have a sense of identity and belonging, shared values, norms, communication, and helping patterns" (Israel, 1985:72).

A "sense of community" is defined and developed as a concept relevant to community organization by various investigators (Allen and Allen, 1990; Chavis et al., 1986; Chavis and Wandersman, 1990; McMillan and Chavis, 1986). Sense of community makes it possible to conceive of a community that crosses geographic boundaries and places. This shared sense of community may unite individuals who are physically dispersed. It is also quite possible to identify with multiple communities that may be physically bound, dispersed, or political in nature. Groups with lower socioeconomic standings, however, are difficult to characterize as to the dominant source of their sense of community. A better understanding of the reference communities of poor and alienated populations may hold clues to the identification of some within them with drug cultures; this phenomenon deserves research attention, both from the standpoint of what causes people to lose their sense of identity with neighborhood communities and from the standpoint of how alternative cultures substitute for the geographic community as a source of social anchoring.

Research on drug abuse prevention in schools often fails to take community structure and dynamics into account. For example, the busing of students to some schools may produce a blended, ungeographically bounded community in the school or a melting pot of community cultures from distinct neighborhoods, each forming a distinct subculture within the school.

Informal political forces often exert more influence on program implementation than the formal political structures associated with official boundaries (Brown, 1984; Rothman and Brown, 1989). Ultimately, the geopolitical scope of a program will be determined by those working in it, guided (in the best case) by local individuals who know the community. The resources available to support the program within the community and from other levels (state or national) are also inportant. As noted in Chapter 1 of this report, disaggregation of community characteristics must be part of any analysis of a culturally diverse population. So too disaggregation of community must also be part of the planning process for programs in order for them to adapt to cultural differences.

Important to the development of drug abuse prevention is the dispersed "community of interest." National advocacy organizations such as the Smoking Control Advocacy Resource Center, Americans for Nonsmokers' Rights, Mothers Against Drunk Driving, the National Association of Prevention Professionals and Advocates all rely on a constituency of concerned citizens scattered around the country. Voluntary and professional associations that advocate and develop prevention initiatives through their networks of members and chapters distributed around the nation represent, in each case, a community of interest. Much of the discussion in this chapter is pertinent to these interest groups on state, national, or international scales (see Paehlke, 1989; Pertschuk and Erikson, 1987; Pertschuk and Schaetzel, 1989; Wallack, 1990).

Although the structural aspect of the definition of community limits activity to a local focus, local community programs are generally coordinated with larger state and national prevention endeavors. Many programs conceived at the national and state levels are designed to be deployed as local community programs. How well these "packaged" community programs can be replicated effectively in multiple, culturally differentiated communities is a question deserving research attention by state and national organizations that sponsor the programs.

In summary, a clear definition of the community involved sets the stage for any research endeavor attempting to understand drug prevention interventions. The meaning and generalizability of such research hinges on which community features are common to other communities and whether these common features are instrumental to the effectiveness of interventions to prevent drug abuse.

Communities and Mass Media

Community-based interventions can be distinguished from interventions carried out at the state or national levels, yet regional- and national-level campaigns can also have a complementary and supportive role in local efforts. (For descriptions of national campaigns sponsored by Public Health Service agencies, including the Office of Substance Abuse Prevention, see Office of Disease Prevention and Health Promotion, 1990.) Where appropriate and feasible, community-based programs try to coordinate their interventions with larger population campaigns to obtain the media benefits as well as other resources that support the larger effort (e.g., Davis and Iverson, 1984; Maloney and Hersey, 1984; Samuels, 1990). Most of the methods used in community media initiatives in prevention programs can be adapted to the state and national levels (see Arkin, 1990; Green et al., 1984; Shoemaker, 1989; Wallack and Atkin, 1990).

The role of the media in communicating substance abuse messages across community boundaries and the effects of bypassing community structures to reach individuals directly, without actively engaging community institutions (e.g., schools, churches, parents), need further research. Both drug-promoting messages (e.g., alcohol advertising, music video entertainment) and antidrug messages (e.g., public service ads) communicated through mass media often reach individuals without institutional screening at the local level (American Medical Association, 1986; Atkin, 1987; 1990; McDonald and Estep, 1985; Wallack et al., 1987). Research is needed not only on the national media depictions of use, but also on the role of community institutions—schools, families, churches, and agencies—in buffering or building on these mass communications.

Besides the mass communications that emanate from outside the community, much use is made in community-wide prevention programs of locally produced or adapted mass communications and local media outlets such as local radio, television, newspapers, and direct mail. These resources are considered in the context of other community interventions in the discussion that follows.

THE LOGIC OF COMMUNITY-WIDE INTERVENTIONS

Much of the prevention research on drug use has been in the specific settings of schools or institutions in contact with high-risk populations, such as juvenile justice divisions. These settings concentrate prevention resources and tailor prevention interventions, affording greater experimental control, greater homogeneity of subject populations, and more certain generalizability of results to similar settings. Nevertheless, there is reason to redirect some program and research efforts toward more community-wide interventions and studies.

Encouraging results from several sources have fostered growing sophistication and larger numbers of community-wide health promotion and disease prevention programs: the large-scale family planning and immunization programs reported in the 1960s and early 1970s (Cuca and Pierce, 1977; Green and McAlister, 1984); antismoking campaigns (Flay, 1987a,b; Warner and Murt, 1983); and cardiovascular and cancer community prevention trials initiated in the late 1970s and early 1980s (Farquhar et al., 1990; Farquhar et al., 1983; Lasater et al., 1984; Nutbeam and Catford, 1987; Puska et al., 1985). The environmental movement has sought a similar level of community-wide activity around issues such as recycling, toxic waste disposal, water conservation, and van pooling (Freudenberg, 1984; Paehlke, 1989; Spretnak and Capra, 1984). The AIDS epidemic, infection with the HIV virus, and teenage pregnancies have revived a parallel and converging interest in community approaches to health education (Becker and Joseph, 1988; Coates et al., 1988; Leviton and Valdiser, 1990; Winett et al., 1990; Markland and Vincent, 1990; McCoy et al., 1990; Ostrow, 1985; Patton, 1985; Williams, 1986). The community-wide approach has the potential of complementing and supporting institution-based programs in three ways: epidemiologic, social psychological, and economical.

Epidemiologic Dimensions

Most community-wide demonstrations are designed to produce small changes in large populations. Numerically speaking, a small percentage change in an entire population would yield greater public health benefits than would a comparable level of effort aimed exclusively at the 10 percent of the population deemed to be at highest risk. More people gain a little, and a little prevention goes a long way relative to a lot of cure, especially when the disease or condition has a contagion aspect to it. Public health analysts provide the epidemiologic and sociological arithmetic justifying these population approaches (Blackburn, 1987; Chamberlin, 1988; Farquhar, 1978; Kottke et al., 1985). Whether these calculations apply when the condition to be prevented is drug use deserves similar epidemiological study. The following studies are examples of how the arithmetic works when the changes sought are behavioral and the outcomes sought are chronic disease reductions.

In a county-wide cardiovascular prevention project in North Karelia, Finland, only 2 percent of the target population lost weight, but this amounted to 60,000 people, far more than could have been reached through doctors' offices (Puska et al., 1981). The Australian Quit For Life media campaign produced a mere 2.8 percent reduction in smoking prevalence (Dwyer et al., 1986; Pierce et al., 1990), which would be considered a failure by targeted smoking cessation program standards (Lando et al., 1990a,b), but it amounted to 83,000 fewer smokers in Sydney. A television and community organization effort to support smokers' quitting in Toronto yielded a 2.9 percent reduction in smoking prevalence, which translated to 8,800 fewer smokers than expected from extrapolated trends in Canada (Millar and Naegele, 1987). The scattered and sporadic but relentless antismoking efforts in the United States between 1964 and 1978 produced a net annual reduction in smoking prevalence of only 1 percent, but this produced in turn an estimated 200,000 fewer premature smoking-related deaths, with many more expected to be avoided as former smokers survive through the 1980s and 1990s (Warner and Murt, 1983). Unlike the programs discussed in Chapters 2 and 3 designed to afffect young, early-phase smokers, these campaigns were addressed primarily to adults with long-established patterns of dependent smoking behavior.

These epidemiologic examples of the extensive, though proportionately small, benefits of community-wide interventions relative to the more effective but limited range of targeted, intensive, institutionally based interventions (Schorr, 1989) argue for a place at the prevention table for community approaches to drug use prevention. Two questions arise, however, in translating the epidemiologic case from disease prevention and health promotion specifically to drug use prevention research. One is whether the prevention of conditions or behaviors that pertain to whole populations, such as the risk of heart disease and related eating behavior, apply in the same ways to prevention of illicit drug abuse prevention. They do apply clearly in the intermediate case of smoking. The other is whether the health implications of small changes in large populations that make the epidemiologic case for health promotion in relation to heart disease and cancer prevention apply to drug use prevention.

Social-Psychological Dimensions

On the basis of their review of decades of research and experience on sexually transmitted disease control, Solomon and DeJong (1986:314) conclude: "More than any other recommendation, we urge that AIDS risk-reduction strategies focus on establishing a social climate in which people feel that it is the norm and not the exception to adopt AIDS risk-reduction behavior." This concept of building a social norm for behavior conducive to health lies at the heart of the social-psychological justification for community approaches to prevention (Dwore and Kreuter, 1980; Green, 1970a,b; Green and McAlister, 1984). Clearly the antismoking initiatives have succeeded in doing just that (Chandler, 1986; Fiore et al., 1989; Flay, 1987a,b; McGinnis et al., 1987; Pierce et al., 1989); designated drivers rather than drinking and driving appear to be making similar strides in becoming a norm (Jernigan and Mosher, 1987; Wallack, 1984); low fat eating has begun to take on the markings of a social norm, at least in more affluent communities and their upscale restaurants (Block et al., 1988; National Restaurant Association, 1989; Popkin et al., 1989; Food Marketing Institute, 1989). The task in these areas, as may be true of drug prevention, appears to be to ensure that such norms diffuse to all segments of the community. This will almost certainly require more targeted research and program efforts in high-risk subpopulations.

However, the social-psychological case does not require choosing between community-wide approaches and targeted approaches. The concept instead is that these approaches may be mutually reinforcing in their effects. Social marketing and classroom learning experience indicate that targeting or "market segmentation" ensures more tailored, relevant, and effective teaching of persuasive messages to individuals (Kotler and Roberto, 1989; Manoff, 1985). But an individual can be powerfully *predisposed* to change his or her own perception that others have made the change successfully (role models) and with satisfaction (vicarious reinforcement). Furthermore, the individual making the change can be *enabled* by imitation and by help from friends, and *reinforced* by the approval of significant others, if enough social change is taking place around the individual, i.e., if other people and environmental circumstances support the change in the same period of time. This is a fundamental thesis of social learning theory (Bandura, 1986; Clark, 1987; Parcel and Baranowski, 1981).

Employing a combination of targeted and community approaches recognizes the reciprocity between individuals and environments and between individualized approaches and system approaches. (For critical reviews of debates that set these approaches against each other rather than on a complementary basis, see Green and Raeburn, 1988; Minkler, 1989; Rimer, 1990; Simons-Morton et al., 1988.) Those undertaking community approaches count on individual innovators to blaze a trail, and also try to reinforce the innovative behavior and reach others by building greater environmental and normative supports. Ordinances to control smoking in public places, for example, give support to those who have quit smoking and protect them from exposure to the smoking behavior of others while also pushing others to quit.

However, research is needed on the potential backlash in some segments of the community when norms are developed through coercive means without effective public education, as when panic about drugs results in massively increased police and other control activity in a community. Such activity alters the social processes in drug-using subcultures (Young, 1981; Courtwright et al., 1989), hardens the boundaries of the subcultural group, and may generate new problems, such as increasingly violent drug dealing.

One theoretical rationale for community programs is to provide environmental and social supports for change through policies and mass media. Another is to coordinate institutional interventions to strengthen psychological readiness or resistance to drugs, through families, schools, work sites, and health care settings, in which more individualized communications can be organized. Policies and mass media, in the long term, help shape psychological readiness, and institutional settings provide ideal opportunities for social and environmental supports for change. In short, the combination of interventions at multiple levels should enhance the diffusion throughout the community necessary to reach indirectly those who are not reached personally directly.

Economic Dimensions

A major barrier to reaching the more economically disadvantaged segments of the population is often the paucity of financial resources available in the poorer parts of the community, where a multitude of problems are concentrated (Oberschall, 1973). Although the drug abuse problem may affect larger numbers of middle-income and more affluent people than poor people, the media tend to portray it as a problem of the poor. Once the parents of adolescents in the middle-income and affluent segments of the community recognize that the problem may well affect their own children, they are more likely to support agencies and programs that reach out to the whole community to prevent the problem. This is the so-called agenda-setting function of mass media and community organization (Gaziano, 1985; Protess et al., 1985; Shaw and McCombs, 1989). Economic and other motives that might underlie public responses to drug problems, such as those revealed in studies of voting behavior and support for school initiatives, need greater attention from the drug abuse prevention research field if school-based programs are to have the support they need from the community to succeed when the researchers are gone.

THE SIZE, SCOPE, AND COMPLEXITY
OF COMMUNITY INTERVENTIONS

Community interventions are more than the sum of multiple interventions in the community. The synergism and leverage sought with the cooperation of several organizations, each with a constituency and a distinct set of resources, requires measures and criteria of process and impact that differ qualitatively as well as quantitatively from those used in research on interventions *in* the community. Community-wide interventions require that the planners have the staff (or at least committed volunteers), resources, and political influence to deliver on the task of involving several sectors of the community, including the major channels of mass communication. Few agencies have the personnel and purview to take on community-wide programs by themselves, and much of the change required in complex issues such as drug abuse prevention calls for broad political support and consensus. For these reasons, *community coalitions* have become the mainstay of most health promotion/disease prevention programs. Despite their popularity, there has been little formal research even to describe the array of coalition types (Couto, 1990), much less to evaluate their efficacy (Feighery and Rogers, 1990). Systematic case studies followed by comparative analyses of different types of coalitions and their effectiveness are very much in order.

From the standpoint of evaluation research, determining the size and scope of community-wide prevention programs depends on having the resources and capacity to collect and analyze the population-based data necessary to detect changes over time. Research is needed on the development of efficient means of data collection and analysis on community norms and behavior related to drug abuse.

The individually small but widespread changes sought by community health programs apply to the majority of the population. Interventions within a community seek more intensive or profound change in a limited subpopulation, usually within or from a specific community site such as the workplace, hospital, clinic, or school. Health care workers using the latter approach can take advantage of the strong reinforcement provided by the group dynamics within institutions and the interpersonal channels of communication. Such interpersonal and small-group interventions are more common, more manageable, and probably better understood than community-wide programs. Institution-based programs lend themselves better to systematic, controlled research, hence their stronger research base. But community-wide programs have greater potential for making significant population changes primarily as a result of reaching larger numbers of people through mass media and multiple channels of communication, building widespread normative, economic, and political support for the changes, and possibly stimulating change in a community's policies and social fabric (Bracht, 1990; Christenson et al., 1989; Green and McAlister, 1984).

Bigger programs are not necessarily better programs. In fact, site- or area-specific health promotion interventions carried out within communities, such as demonstration programs in schools, have provided the strongest evidence of short-term impact and flexibility to. adapt to the special needs of subpopulations and individuals, and they can serve as models and inspirations for broader community change by other organizations that will emulate them (Carlaw et al., 1984; Green et al., 1991; Orlandi et al., 1990). As more organizations adopt or extend components of the program, a multiplier effect gets under way, with the funded demonstration projects being emulated by others without external funding (Kreuter et al., 1982). Research on examples of the diffusion or multiplier effect of drug abuse prevention projects should be possible, considering, for example, the number of community demonstration projects being funded by the Center for Substance Abuse Prevention grants.

APPROACHES TO COMMUNITY-BASED RESEARCH

Community Participation

The larger the community, the greater will be the number of representatives of subcommunities and cooperating organizations engaged in the planning for community-wide interventions. Early involvement of community members in identifying their own needs, setting their own priorities, and planning their own programs is in itself an intervention. It provides the opportunity for ownership that can lead to a sense of empowerment and self-determination.

Gaining broad-based community participation for the federally funded, large-scale research and demonstration efforts in prevention, however, has been problematic. Up-front community initiation and participation in the pioneering community intervention trials in family planning, heart disease prevention, and cancer control has been limited, for good reason. These large scientific studies were conceived and, for the most part, planned by public health officials at the federal level and professors who received the research grants or contracts. Efforts to engage the community typically occurred after the planning had been started, if not completed. The protocol was approved by a national peer review panel and the grant approved by a federal agency. The active participation of the community could usually come only after the grant was in hand. Asking communities and organizations to implement programs planned elsewhere and evaluated on someone else's terms might gain some followers, but the duration of their commitment may be only for "as long as the money lasts."

Researchers working on large community interventions face a paradox. They must design the proposals for scientific trials and rigorously evaluated demonstrations according to guidelines of the federal government. Community participation thus begins when key people in the target communities are informed of the researcher's intent to apply for the grant and their willingness to cooperate is needed for the application. This form of community participation may be criticized as too little, too late. If community leaders are invited to participate in the implementation but not in the policy and planning stages, they may feel they are being used as free labor for university-initiated projects. This dilemma reflects an inability to design unbiased scientific tests of community interventions without damaging a variable (active community participation) that is likely to be essential for successful community structural and cultural change, as well as behavioral change in individuals (Green, 1977; Holder and Giesbrecht, 1989). Very early activation of the community in these instances may falsely raise community hopes and expectations should funding not be secured. Nevertheless, some communities go on from this point to develop their own programs without external funding. Pentz and her colleagues (1986) have attempted (with mixed success) to address some of these issues in balancing program and research integrity in Project STAR, the Midwestern Prevention Project.

The scientific benefits of the early community studies may have justified their restraints on early and active participation of community members. The evidence pointing to the benefits of community participation (Bracht and Kingsbury, 1990; Green, 1986; Hunt, 1990; Minkler, 1990) now demands a continuing search for funding mechanisms between levels of government and procedures of grant making that provide for greater community involvement (Green, 1986; Williams, 1990).

Program Implementation and Evaluation

Much of the success or failure of programs imitating or attempting to replicate previously demonstrated and evaluated prevention programs can be attributed to the quality and performance of management, personnel, and resources deployed to implement the program. A growing body of literature on the evaluation of implementation, or process evaluation, has developed in recent years (King et al., 1987; Ottoson and Green, 1987; Reid and Hanrahan, 1988). Considering the wide variety of personnel implementing drug abuse prevention programs as well as the rapid development of new strategies, further research on implementation problems and evaluations of implementation must be supported.

Training and Evaluation

The Office of Substance Abuse Prevention spends some $30 million annually on training. Upgrading the skills of personnel working in drug abuse prevention is necessitated by the fast-breaking results of research and evaluation on new innovations in prevention programming. Training, like program implementation, has been relatively neglected as an object of research and evaluation in all fields of prevention until recent years, but a growing literature is taking shape (Easterby-Smith, 1986; Fitz-enz, 1984; Phillips, 1983; Staropoli and Waltz, 1978). Most of the published work on the evaluation of training has been in the form of exhortations to practitioners to do more of it and manuals to help them do so. Serious development of measurement tools and standardization of criteria for the evaluation of training needs support (Battista and Mickalide, 1990; Brinkerhoff, 1987).

Diffusion Research

Once research indicates the feasibility, effectiveness, and generalizability of specific interventions in specific settings, the next level of research and evaluation should assess ways to facilitate the diffusion of these innovative strategies. The National Cancer Institute, the National Institute for Dental Research, and the National Heart, Lung, and Blood Institute are now supporting such diffusion research on the site-specific (school, clinical, and workplace) adoption of interventions for prevention that have been tested in previous field or clinical trials (Basch, 1984; Basch et al., 1986; Brunk and Goeppinger, 1990; Coombs et al., 1981; Orlandi, 1986; Orlandi et al., 1990; Parcel et al., 1989a,b; Portnoy et al., 1989; Scheirer, 1990). Similar research on the diffusion of drug abuse prevention innovations is likely to yield similar conclusions about the correlates of successful diffusion and adoption, but the research needs to be sponsored and completed before this assumption can be accepted.

Community-Wide Trials

The need for developmental and outcome studies on the proliferating community-wide programs is urgent; these projects are based on the logic and theoretical foundations outlined above, but their efficacy in preventing drug abuse can only be inferred at this time from a handful of studies in family planning, immunization, smoking, and cardiovascular risk reduction. The closest a National Institute on Drug Abuse (NIDA) project has come to verifying community organization models derived from other fields is in the Midwestern Prevention Project (Pentz, 1986; Pentz et al., 1986); the data reported to date, however, are based only on the school-based component of the program in one city, with parental involvement and mass media coverage (Pentz et al., 1989). NIDA might have tested the viability and efficacy of community coalitions for drug abuse prevention before they were announced as a required component of grants from the Department of Health and Human Services.

The National Institute on Alcohol Abuse and Alcoholism (NIAAA) sponsored a conference on Methodological Issues in Community Prevention Trials for Alcohol Problems at the University of California, Berkeley, in December 1989 (Holder, 1991). Drawing on the experience of the recently completed community trials in cardiovascular risk reduction funded by the National Heart, Lung, and Blood Institute, the papers presented at that conference brought out many of the same methodological differences and similarities that face research on community-wide strategies for drug abuse prevention.

SCHOOL AS A SETTING FOR INTERVENTION

Most of the drug abuse prevention research, as seen in the chapters of this report, has been conducted in school settings. We believe the issues in the use of the school as a setting for drug abuse prevention center as much on the conflict of purposes and the proper use and preparation of teachers as on the specific content of methods of intervention. Drug abuse prevention in schools must depend for its administrative acceptance and support on the ability to demonstrate an impact on *educational* goals, not just on drug use or abuse.

Purpose and Functions of School Health Programs

Those concerned about drug abuse sometimes promote the health or social objectives of prevention without much apparent attention to the priorities of cooperating organizations. Nowhere do these differences between the perspectives of those representing different sectors clash more than in school health. From the health perspective, schools represent a valuable resource for drug abuse prevention, but schools are relatively independent of the health and social service sectors.

Every school day nearly 47 million students attend elementary and secondary schools in the United States; about 6 million professional and other workers staff those schools. (American Council of Life Insurance, 1985). (The numbers and proportion of school-based staff is larger if one includes colleges, universities, and the rapidly growing number of preschool and day care centers. The principles discussed here apply similarly in college drug abuse prevention programs.) Schools thus constitute the center of activity for nearly one-fifth of the U.S. population. Orchestrated drug abuse prevention in schools might constitute society's most cost-effective prevention strategy (Carnegie Council on Adolescent Development, 1989).

From the educator's perspective the school has a different set of priorities, and many believe its educational role in society should not be compromised in the pursuit of health or drug abuse prevention objectives. Some argue that even behavioral objectives, including health behavior, have no place in the school's mission because they detract from the primary objectives of learning critical thinking and reasoning (Resnick, 1987). The most acceptable justification of drug abuse prevention and health services in the school has been to ensure that students would be kept healthy enough and attentive enough to be able to attend and benefit from school activities (Kolbe et al., 1986).

School personnel need the cooperation and resources of community agencies and media in support of the school's mission, especially when that mission is expanded to include purposes such as drug abuse prevention that go beyond the school's educational mandate. Students spend one-third of their work-week hours in school, but they spend more than two-thirds of total hours, counting weekends, holidays, and summer vacations, outside the school. Furthermore, some of the children and youth who need help with drug abuse prevention the most have dropped out of school or have such high absenteeism that they will not be reached by school programs. Schools alone cannot solve society's health and social problems. They tend to sidestep the responsibility to address problems such as drug abuse as long as they perceive their own educational role as threatened by the siphoning of the school's resources into areas they consider tangential to their basic educational mission (Kolbe and Iverson, 1983).

The educational priorities of schools become even more compelling for school personnel when budgets are tight (as they have been for decades) and when parents and employers become concerned about the decline in student performance on standardized tests in reading, writing, and arithmetic. The back-to-basics pressures on schools tend to push health education, physical education, and even school nursing services into the background, signaling a perception of their diminished status (Allanson, 1978; Hertel, 1982; Kolbe, 1982). Yet there is growing evidence of the benefits of these elements and services for school-age children in reducing absenteeism, increasing average daily attendance, improving attentiveness, reducing vandalism, and other aspects of the school's mission (Kolbe et al., 1986).

Components of School Health

The basic structure of school health programs as reflected in the literature has remained relatively unchanged for over 50 years. It consists of three interdependent components: (1) health instruction, (2) school health services, and (3) a healthful school environment (Cornacchia et al., 1988; Creswell and Newman, 1989; Pollock and Middleton, 1989).

Comprehensive school health refers to these multiple components of the school health program within the school as well as the active involvement of parents and the community in the health affairs of the school and on behalf of the health of school-age children (Becker et al., 1989; Perry et al., 1988). *Comprehensive school health education* refers to an instructional program that provides for an integrated, K-12 curriculum covering the full range of health topics and problems. Such comprehensive approaches have gained considerable credence and acceptability with school administrators and teachers in preference to "disease-of-the-year" approaches that have tended to create curricular chaos as federal and state categorical funding changes too frequently to permit an integrated program. Add to this the virtual barrage of categorical curricula that each voluntary association seeks to introduce into the school and one can appreciate the school's strong preference for a single comprehensive approach.

A new generation of school-based studies on drug abuse prevention might be in order. Such research could examine the role of drug topics within the context of the comprehensive school health curriculum; the role of the curriculum (instructional component) within the context of school health services and environment; and the role of the school within the context of a network of other community resources and channels of communication to determine how the school programs in drug abuse prevention complement other community efforts.

Evaluation of School Health Education

After decades of basing support for comprehensive school health on learning principles and research evidence borrowed from other fields, contemporary school health literature is suddenly endowed with rigorous evaluations of well-designed school health and school health education programs. The most sweeping evidence, contributed to the literature in the 1980s, was the nationwide evaluation of the comprehensive School Health Curriculum Project. From a handful of small-scale studies conducted before 1980 with limited controls (usually pretest-posttest designs) and with little behavioral impact measured (usually knowledge and attitude changes only—see Green et al., 1980), the opportunity arose in 1981 to carry out a multisite randomized evaluation of this project and several other health curricula with support from the U.S. Office of Disease Prevention and Health Promotion and the Centers for Disease Control.

The School Health Education Evaluation was a pioneering 3-year prospective study, involving 30,000 students in grades 4-7 in 20 states. It revealed that students who were exposed to comprehensive school health education not only showed significant positive changes in their health-related knowledge and attitudes, compared with students in matched schools without such exposure, but they were also considerably less likely to take up smoking. Especially relevant were those findings that clearly demonstrated that administrative support and teacher training were directly linked to the positive student outcomes detected, as were the cumulative number of hours of classroom time devoted to comprehensive school health education (Connell et al., 1985; Connell and Turner, 1985; Cook and Walberg, 1985; Gunn et al., 1985; Olsen et al., 1985; Owen et al., 1985).

The National Institutes of Health has commissioned several panels of scientists to review what has been learned about school health education (e.g., Kreuter and Reagan, 1980; Newman, 1980; O'Rourke and Stone, 1980; Kolbe and Iverson, 1980; Kolbe et al., 1986). In 1988, an expert advisory group convened by the National Cancer Institute (NCI) reviewed 20 years of research on school-based efforts to prevent tobacco use. The panel found nine areas with sufficient data or experience to reach preliminary conclusions and recommendations: program, impact, focus, context, length, ideal age for intervention, teacher training, program implementation, and the need for peer and parental involvement (Glynn, 1989, describes the 15 school-based smoking prevention studies supported by NCI; in the same issue, eight studies of smokeless tobacco prevention trials supported by NCI are described by Boyd and Glover, 1989; the American Cancer Society's and NCI's development and evaluation of a school nutrition and cancer education curriculum is described in Light and Contento, 1989).

The National Heart, Lung, and Blood Institute supported a variety of school-based research efforts, 10 of which are summarized in Table A.1 (Stone et al., 1989). As the table indicates, these studies reflect diversity in the demographic characteristics of the populations studied, the risk factor focus, and the methods and channels of intervention. Several of the studies emphasized the importance of a planning model to complement and organize specific theoretical models (Best, 1989). As a result, this collection of studies placed rather strong emphasis on the home to address reinforcing factors in the social environment as a complement to school interventions.

A panel convened by the Kaiser Family Foundation concluded that drug abuse prevention programs are likely be most effective when implemented in the context of comprehensive school health programs linked with community health promotion programs (Flay, 1986; Pentz, 1986; Perry, 1986).

The Family as a Channel

The studies summarized in Table A.1 are identified as school-based studies, but 7 of the 10 use the strategy of linking home and school as mutually reinforcing settings for children's behavior. In the Nader et al. study (1989), the family is the primary locus or channel of change rather than the school and its environment, which serve a supportive role.

Efforts to expand the focus of school programs to place increasing emphasis on the home and family are supported by findings from a 1988 national school health education survey sponsored by the Metropolitan Life Foundation (1988). The survey sampled over 4,000 students from 199 public schools and 500 randomly selected parents of children attending schools. Among other things, the survey revealed that, while the majority of both teachers and parents believe that parental involvement in children's health education would be of considerable help in encouraging good health habits for children, most parents (71 percent) report never getting involved in the process. Lack of parental involvement may in part explain why parents do not know the extent of drinking, smoking, or drug-taking by their children. Whereas 36 percent of the parents surveyed indicated that their child has had at least one alcoholic drink, 66 percent of the students said they had alcohol at least once or twice; only 14 percent of parents reported that their child had smoked a cigarette, whereas 41 percent of students said they had smoked; 5 percent of parents said that their child had used drugs, whereas 17 percent of students reported having used drugs.

International investigators have also conducted studies that employ close collaboration among key institutions within the community and with the family. The North Karelia, Finland, Youth Project included modifications in the school diet, health screening, mass media, comprehensive school health education, and parental support to reduce the major risk factors for noncommunicable diseases. Findings after two years revealed decreases in smoking and alcohol use in the randomized intervention schools compared with eight randomized reference schools (Vartiainen et al., 1986).

The common denominators for these successful programs and others like them include: (1) a commitment to addressing specific problems or modifiable risk factors, often within the context of a comprehensive approach and (2) the use of multiple intervention methods based on an assessment of the characteristics, needs, and interests of the target population and designed to reach the individual through multiple channels including media, institutions, and the individual's family and peer groups.

Questions for further research to make these findings pertinent to drug abuse prevention are whether the behavioral changes with respect to tobacco and alcohol, among others, respond to different interventions or different channels of communication than do illicit drug behaviors; and whether these findings can be generalized to the ethnic and school dropout populations of high-risk youth. In general, the preventive approaches that have been rigorously evaluated would require one-size-fits-all assumptions in order to be generalized to drug abusing and ethnic groups other than those in which they have been tested. Research on the relationships among problem behaviors and preventive or risk-avoiding behaviors in children suggest a clustering of problem behaviors (Donovan and Jessor, 1985) and health-

TABLE A.1 Summary of NHLBI School-Based Health Promotion Studies

Investigator Institution Study	Ethnicity[a] SES Grade State	Schools[b] Classes Students	Curr Food Home	Provider	Target Areas	Outcomes
Perry, Cheryl University of Minnesota "Healthy Heart" "The Home Team"	W,A SES (M) Grade 3 MN, ND	24T/7C 1405/T 422C	Curr Home	Teachers Mail	Eating	Changes in knowledge, total fat, saturated fat, complex carbohydrate intake
Parcel, Guy University of Texas "Go For Health"	W,H,B SES (L,M) Grades 3-4 TX	2T/2C 40 1156	Curr Food Serv	Teachers Food Workers	Eating Exercise	Changes in knowledge, self-efficacy, behavioral expectations food serv, PE classes, diet
Walter, Heather American Health Fdn "Know Your Body"	W,B,A,H SES (L,M,H) Grades 4-9 NY	22T/15C 2075T 1313C	Curr Home	Teachers	Eating Exercise Smoking BP WT	Changes in knowledge, total fat, complex carbohydrate intake, cholesterol, initiation of smoking
Bush, Patricia Georgetown University "Know Your Body"	B SES (L,M,H) Grades 4-9 DC	6T/3C 707T 334C	Curr Home	Teachers	Eating Exercise Smoking BP WT	Changes in knowledge, smoking attitudes, BP, HDL cholesterol, fitness, thiocyanate
Nader, Philip University of CA-SD "Family Health Project"	H,W SES (L,M) Grades 5-6 CA	6T/6C 163T 160C	Home	Inst	Eating Exercise	Changes in diet, cholesterol, BP, knowledge

Study	Population	N	Setting	Agent	Behaviors	Outcomes
Cohen, Rita Brownell, Kelly University of Penn "CV Risk Reduction"	W SES (M) Grades 5-7 PA	1062T 992C	Curr Home	Teachers Peers	Eating BP Smoking	Changes in knowledge, initiation of smoking, peers were equally or more effective than teachers
Fors, Stuart, Univ of Georgia "3R's + HBP"	W,B SES (L,M) Grade 6 GA	14T/7C 60 853T 351C	Curr Home	Teachers Students	BP	Changes in knowledge, taking BP
Ellison, R. Curtis University of Mass "Food Service Project"	W,B,A SES (M,H) Grade 9 MA, NH	2 1100	Food Serv	Food Workers	BP Eating	Changes in BP, cholesterol, and food service
Weinberg, Armin Baylor College of Med "CV Curr/Family Tree"	W,H,B SES (L,M) Grades 9-10 TX	7 40 5787	Curr Home	Teachers	Eating Exercise BP	Changes in knowledge, attitudes, self-report beh., parents used smoking + wt + exercise
Killen, Joel Farquhar, John Stanford Univ "CV Risk Reduction"	W,H,A SES (M) Grade 10 CA	2T/2C 8 1447	Curr	Inst	Eating Exercise BP Smoking	Changes in knowledge, exercise, smoking, resting heart rate, BMI, skinfolds

NOTE: All work cited appears in *Health Education Quarterly* 16(2).

[a]Predominant ethnic/racial group: A, Asian; B, Black; H, Hispanic; W, White.
[b]T, treatment; C, control.

SOURCE: Stone et al. (1989:160-161).

related behaviors (Terre et al., 1990), but the clusters may vary with age. These findings make the assumption of the appropriateness of similar one-size-fits-all approaches partially supportable and partly questionable.

THE WORKPLACE SETTING

This report does not deal specifically with drug abuse prevention programs in the workplace; a separate National Research Council committee is conducting a multidimensional study of workplace drug programs (National Research Council, 1993). Nevertheless, as a potential channel of communication on drug abuse prevention and a setting for related programs, the workplace merits some mention here. Workplaces are to adults as schools are to children: a place where they spend many of their waking hours, where group affiliations are shaped, where rewards are received for performance and productivity. It is also a place where many adult users maintain access to drugs and where strong leverage can be exercised through the threat of job loss.

About three-fourths of adult men (age 16 and over) and over half of adult women in the United States are in the labor force (Bureau of the Census, 1989). The increase in the female work force participation rate, especially working mothers, is reshaping the attitudes of employers toward employee benefits and working conditions. The workplace has replaced the neighborhood as the community of reference and social identity for many urban and suburban North Americans and Europeans (see, for example, Duhl, 1986; Glynn, 1981; Green, 1990; Riger and Lavraka, 1981).

These demographic and social trends, combined with the pervasive influence of occupational environments on adult health, quality of life, behavior and lifestyle, make work sites logical settings for preventive approaches to drug abuse. As with other settings, the example of other health promotion initiatives provides hypotheses for research and potential models for drug abuse prevention.

Yet, more than other settings, workplaces have failed to incorporate drug abuse prevention in their health promotion programs. Based on secondary analyses of a survey sponsored by NIDA, Cook and Harrell (1987:358) concluded:

> If drug abuse prevention is to be found in industry, one might expect to find it within the growing number of health promotion programs in the workplace, programs that emphasize the development of healthful practices through preventive means. Yet an examination of even the most comprehensive health promotion programs (e.g. the programs at Johnson and Johnson, Control Data and AT&T), reveals that drug and alcohol prevention is not a part of these efforts.

Given this paucity of substance abuse prevention in the context of pro-liferating workplace health promotion programs, a brief look at the research on industry incentives for adopting health promotion programs may be in-structive. American business and industry took a fresh look at health pro-motion and disease prevention in the late 1970s as they faced the opening waves of alarming increases in the cost of medical care and insurance pre-miums for their employees (Collings, 1982). In 1990, employers paid $186.2 billion or approximately 29 percent of all expenditures for personal health care services and supplies in the United States (Levit and Cowan, 1991). Employers began to initiate health promotion programs based on a growing awareness of their potential health and economic benefits (Fielding, 1982; Fielding and Breslow, 1983; Parkinson and Associates, 1982). Through repeated exposures to health messages via a myriad of formal and informal communication channels, the general public, including employers, began to see the relevance of the information confirming the link between health and factors they had the power to change.

Although industry has responded with substantial commitments to new initiatives in workplace health promotion, the drug abuse issue has been addressed almost entirely within a treatment (employee assistance program) and enforcement (drug testing) framework rather than one of prevention. The health promotion programs themselves, especially the fitness and stress management programs, can be seen as primary prevention of drug abuse. Evaluation of these and other health promotion and employee assistance programs, based on a survey of 550 corporations (Katzman and Smith, 1989), has been extremely limited. Only 41 out of the 98 respondent firms reported that they were currently evaluating their programs, and most of these were using nonexperimental methods. Workplace health promotion appears to be today about where school health education was in 1980 with respect to rigor of research evaluation. Considering their potential for ef-fective drug abuse prevention, workplace programs deserve much more re-search attention than they have been given.

THE HEALTH CARE SETTING

As we have seen, considerable attention has been directed to drug abuse preventive interventions delivered in the school setting, usually by teachers, sometimes supplemented by peers of the students receiving the instruction. Research on drug use prevention in the school setting has overshadowed the limited prevention research in medical care settings. This setting, however, has had a lively development of research on interventions to prevent other problems besides illegal drug use (Cohen, 1979; Haynes et al., 1979; Lawrence, 1990; Matarazzo et al., 1984; Mechanic, 1983; Mullen and Zapka, 1982).

In many communities, health care professionals, particularly physicians, are relied on as the local experts on the abuse of alcohol and drugs; others, however—nurses, pharmacists, dentists, and other professionals—offer equally attractive settings and channels through which to reach people at risk of drug abuse and to deliver preventive interventions.

The medical, dental, nursing, or pharmaceutical setting has the potential to provide prevention of substance abuse through patient counseling on the hazards of drugs; this is most likely to occur when a problem already appears to be present. Very little research on primary prevention counseling on drug abuse has been carried out in such settings (U.S. Preventive Services Task Force, 1989).

One criterion that should be used in determining who will deliver what preventive interventions and what settings deserve greater research focus is the potential coverage of segments of the population most needing the intervention. A second criterion is available time to deliver the intervention. A third criterion is credibility with the recipients.

Dentists and dental offices, for example, meet all three criteria of potential coverage, available time, and credibility. Dentists have credibility within communities as health professionals. They spend substantial amounts of time with their patients; a normal office visit includes at least 30 minutes with the dentist and often an additional 30 minutes with a dental hygienist. Dentists are less specialized and more prevention-oriented than physicians and see their patients on a more consistent schedule; 63 percent of Americans report at least one visit with their dentist each year, and the annual number of visits to the dentist per patient averages 2. Of greater significance from a prevention perspective, dentists often treat entire families rather than isolated and independent individuals.

Dental offices are good settings for drug abuse prevention because cigarettes, smokeless tobacco products, and other drugs that are smoked (e.g., marijuana, cocaine) can be readily detected. The first evidence of use of these products by young people who would not admit their use may be in the oral cavity. The oral tissue is assaulted by both the hot smoke as well as the particulate matter in these drug delivery systems. In the case of smokeless tobacco, there are exceedingly high levels of carcinogenic nitrosomines in each package. Dentists closely examine the affected oral tissues and can readily detect the effects of use with normal observations (Greene et al., 1990). The hygienist can be trained to provide a booster to the intervention provided by the dentist as well as supplemental skill training for maintaining healthy oral tissue.

A particular category accessible through health care settings are people who medicate themselves by taking drugs for an illness, who risk making a variety of mistakes, including use of an inappropriate drug, the wrong dosage of the right drug, or the right drug at the wrong time. The most blatant form of drug abuse in this category is self-administration of larger doses of psychotropic drugs than prescribed and continued use beyond the prescribed period. Public education through nonmedical channels can reach most consumers to warn them about these potential hazards (National Research Council, 1989). Research on these aspects of drug abuse prevention warrant particular attention considering the number of people at risk.

SUMMARY

Much has been published from the extensive research on selective use of various settings and channels for prevention in areas other than drug abuse. The development of drug abuse prevention research need not repeat all of these studies to ensure that their results are applicable to the specific problems of preventing drug abuse. Many of the research furrows plowed by investigators in family planning, communicable disease control, chronic disease control, and alcohol abuse prevention have proved to be unfruitful and so need not be repeated with drug abuse prevention. But a more systematic examination of the commonalities and differences between drug abuse prevention programs and those of other areas would advance the field of drug abuse prevention more rapidly than an isolated research agenda that seeks to build only on prior research within the sphere of drug abuse etiology and prevention programs.

Most of the prevention research, in all but the school setting, has been in fields other than drug abuse. Within the schools, drug abuse prevention research would do well to link its program innovations and trials with more comprehensive curricula and school-community efforts. Those related to smoking prevention, teenage pregnancy prevention, and dropout prevention share similar methods and goals. School administrators will be more likely to adopt and maintain a curriculum that covers all of these problems comprehensively than to have to construct each element individually. This integrative approach is already working for other areas of school education.

Community-wide programs that include mass media and multiple settings have been relatively neglected as an object of systematic research in drug abuse. Other fields, particularly cardiovascular disease prevention, have much to offer from their extensive community trials.

Two main themes stand out from the review undertaken in this appendix. First, it is critical to learn what constitutes the communities that are relevant to drug abuse prevention. What normative symbols, practices, events, and institutions do those at risk, and those who can influence them, identify with and respond to? How do drug-specific norms and behaviors dovetail with other health norms and behaviors? These questions are particularly salient in low-income areas where assumptions that are built into public programs—assumptions about family stability and support, membership in voluntary associations, literacy, commitments to core institutions, levels of safety—become uncertain. Richly grained, systematic community studies using qualitative and quantitative methods were at one time a thriving research enterprise that contributed to the formation of public policies on health and welfare and the shaping of specific programs to carry out public purposes, neighborhood by neighborhood.

NIDA is not in a position to support a study of every community in the country, nor are the research resources available for this. NIDA is, however, in a position to launch a strategic community research initiative: a research program to develop in a significant number of locations comprehensive assays of community norms, identity, structure, and potentials for prevention coalition-building, based on the presence, absence, or levels of effectiveness of key services and institutions—including schools, workplaces, and health care settings—that can serve as platforms for sustained prevention efforts. Such study sites can become laboratories for developing community models and testing study methodologies that may be practicable for every locality to use.

The urgency of the drug problem in U.S. policy has driven many new drug abuse prevention programs into the field without much research. This has forced the recognition that some of the interventions and their specifications rest on assumptions of efficacy and effectiveness based on generalizations from other fields of prevention in which they have been tested. This is notably the case with respect to research on issues of implementation and sustainability of programs. For example, the "community partnership" grants of OSAP require the applicants to have community coalitions. This requirement is based on strictly anecdotal experience from drug abuse prevention projects, and a little research on coalitions in other fields.

A second major concern is that the study of how comprehensive programs that incorporate drug prevention are implemented; how training is carried out, with what effect on trainee attitudes, knowledge, and behavior; and how concepts and findings are diffused or disseminated.

REFERENCES

Abrams, D.B., J.P. Elder, R.A. Carleton, T.M. Lasater, and L.M. Artz
    1986   Social learning principles for organizational health promotion: an integrated approach. Pp. 28-51 in M.F. Cataldo and T.J. Coates, eds., *Health and Industry: A Behavioral Medicine Perspective*. New York: John Wiley.
Allanson, J.F.
    1978   School nursing services: some current justifications and cost-benefit implications. *Journal of School Health* 48:603-607.
Allen, J., and R.F. Allen
    1990   A sense of community, a shared vision and a positive culture: core enabling factors in successful culture-based change. Pp. 5-18 in R.D. Patton and W.B. Cissel, eds., *Community Organization: Traditional Principles and Modern Applications*. Johnson City, Tenn.: Latchpins Press.

American Council of Life Insurance
  1985   *Wellness at the School Worksite: A Manual.* Washington, D.C.: Health Insurance Association of America.
American Medical Association
  1986   Alcohol advertising, counteradvertising, and depiction in the public media. *Journal of the American Medical Association* 256:1485-1488.
Arkin, E.B.
  1990   Opportunities for improving the nation's health through collaboration with the mass media. *Public Health Reports* 105:219-223.
Atkin, C.
  1987   Alcoholic-beverage advertising: its content and impact. *Advances in Substance Abuse* 1(Suppl.):267-287.
Atkin, C.K.
  1990   Effects of televised alcohol messages on teenage drinking patterns. *Journal of Adolescent Health Care* 11(1):10-24.
Bandura, A.
  1986   *Social Foundations of Thought and Action: A Social Cognitive Theory.* Englewood Cliffs: Prentice Hall.
Basch, C.E.
  1984   Research on disseminating and implementing health education programs in schools. (Proceedings of the National Heart, Lung, Blood Institute Conference on School Health Research) *Journal of School Health* 54:57-66.
Basch, C.E., J.D. Eveland, and B. Portnoy
  1986   Diffusion systems for education and learning about health. *Family and Community Health* 9(2):1-26.
Battista, R.N., and A.D. Mickalide
  1990   Integration of preventive services into primary care: a conceptual framework for implementation. Pp. 467-473 in R.B. Goldbloom and R.S. Lawrence, eds., *Preventing Disease: Beyond the Rhetoric.* New York: Springer-Verlag.
Becker, M.H., and J. Joseph
  1988   AIDS and behavioral change to reduce risk: a review. *American Journal of Public Health* 78:394-410.
Becker, S.L., J.A. Burke, R.A. Arbogast, M.J. Naughton, I. Bachman, and E. Spohn
  1989   Community programs to enhance in-school anti-tobacco efforts. *Preventive Medicine* 18:221-228.
Best, J.A.
  1989   Intervention perspectives on school health promotion research. *Health Education Quarterly* 16:299-306.
Blackburn, H.
  1987   Research and demonstration projects in community cardiovascular disease prevention. *Journal of Public Health Policy* 4:398-421.
Block, G., W. Rosenberger, and B. Patterson
  1988   Calories, fat and cholesterol: intake patterns in the U.S. population by race, sex and age. *American Journal of Public Health* 78:1150.
Boyd, G.M., and E.D. Glover
  1989   Smokeless tobacco use by youth in the U.S. *Journal of School Health* 59:189-194.
Bracht, N., ed.
  1990   *Health Promotion at the Community Level.* Newbury Park, Calif.: Sage.
Bracht, N., and L. Kingsbury
  1990   Community organization principles in health promotion: a five-stage model. Pp. 66-88 in N. Bracht, ed., *Health Promotion at the Community Level.* Newbury Park, Calif.: Sage.

Breckon, D.J., J.R. Harvey, and R.B. Lancaster
1989   *Community Health Education: Settings, Roles, and Skills*, 2nd ed. Rockville, Md.: Aspen.

Brinkerhoff, R.O.
1987   *Achieving Results from Training: How to Evaluate Human Resource Development to Strengthen Programs and Increase Impact.* San Francisco: Jossey-Bass Publishers.

Brown, E.R.
1984   Community organization influence on local public health care policy: a general research model and comparative case study. *Health Education Quarterly* 10:205-234.

Brunk, S.E., and J. Goeppinger
1990   Process evaluation: assessing re-invention of community-based interventions. *Evaluation and the Health Professions* 13:186-203.

Bureau of the Census
1989   *Statistical Abstract of the United States: 1990*, 109th ed. Washington, D.C.: U.S. Government Printing Office.

Carlaw, R.W., M. Mittlemark, N. Bracht, and R. Luepker
1984   Organization for a community cardiovascular health program: experiences from the Minnesota Heart Health Program. *Health Education Quarterly* 11:243-252.

Carnegie Council on Adolescent Development
1989   *Turning Points: Preparing American Youth for the 21st Century.* New York: Carnegie Corporation.

Chamberlin, R.W., ed.
1988   *Beyond Individual Risk Assessment: Community Wide Approaches to Promoting the Health and Development of Families and Children.* Washington, D.C.: National Center for Education in Maternal and Child Care.

Chandler, W.U.
1986   *Worldwatch Paper 68: Banishing Tobacco.* Washington, D.C.: Worldwatch Institution.

Chavis, D.M., and A. Wandersman
1990   Sense of community in the urban environment: a catalyst for participation and community development. *American Journal of Community Psychology* 18:55-81.

Chavis, D.M., J.H. Hogge, D.W. McMillan, and A. Wandersman
1986   Sense of community through Brunswik's lens: a first look. *Journal of Community Psychology* 14:24-40.

Christenson, J.A., K. Fendley, and J.W. Robinson, Jr., eds.
1989   *Community Development in Perspective.* Ames: Iowa State University Press.

Clark, N.M.
1987   Social learning theory in current health education practice. Pp. 251-275 in W.B. Ward, ed., *Advances in Health Education and Promotion*, Vol. 2. Greenwich, Conn.: JAI Press Inc.

Coates, T., R. Stall, and C. Hoff
1988   *Changes in High Risk Behavior Among Gay and Bisexual Men Since the Beginning of the AIDS Epidemic.* Washington, D.C.: Office of Technology Assessment, U.S. Congress.

Cohen, S., ed.
1979   *New Directions in Patient Compliance.* Lexington, Mass.: Lexington Books, D.C. Heath.

Collings, G.H., Jr.
1982   Perspectives of industry regarding health promotion. Pp. 119-126 in R.S. Parkinson and Associates, *Managing Health Promotion in the Workplace: Guidelines for Implementation and Evaluation.* Palo Alto, Calif.: Mayfield Publishing Co.

Connell, D.B., and R.R. Turner
  1985   The impact of instructional experience and the effects of cumulative instruction. *Journal of School Health* 55:324-331.
Connell, D.B., R.R. Turner, and E.F. Mason
  1985   Summary findings of the school health education evaluation: health promotion effectiveness, implementation and costs. *Journal of School Health* 55:316-32.
Cook, R., and A. Harrell
  1987   Drug abuse among working adults: prevalence rates and recommended strategies. *Health Education Research* 2:353-359.
Cook, T.D., and H.J. Walberg
  1985   Methodological and substantive significance. *Journal of School Health* 55:340-343.
Coombs, J.A., J.B. Silversin, E.M. Rogers, and M.E. Drolette
  1981   The transfer of preventive health technologies to schools: a focus on implementation. *Social Science and Medicine* 15A:789-799.
Cornacchia, H.J., L.K. Olsen, and C.J. Nickerson
  1988   *Health in Elementary Schools*, 7th ed. St. Louis, Mo.: Times Mirror/Mosby College Publishing.
Courtwright, D., H. Joseph, and D. Des Jarlais
  1989   *Addicts Who Survived: An Oral History of Narcotic Use in America, 1923-1965.* Knoxville: University of Tennessee.
Couto, R.A.
  1990   Promoting health at the grass roots. *Health Affairs* 9(2):144-151.
Creswell, W.H., and I.M. Newman
  1989   *School Health Practice*, 9th ed. St.Louis, Mo.: Times Mirror/Mosby.
Cuca, R., and C.S. Pierce
  1977   *Experiments in Family Planning: Lessons from the Developing World.* Baltimore, Md.: Johns Hopkins University Press.
Davis, M.F., and D.C. Iverson
  1984   An overview and analysis of the Health Style Campaign. *Health Education Quarterly* 11:253-272.
Dignan, M., and P. Carr
  1986   *Program Planning for Health Education and Health Promotion.* Philadelphia, Pa.: Lea and Febiger.
Donovan, J.E., and R. Jessor
  1985   Structure of problem behavior in adolescence and young adulthood. *Journal of Consulting and Clinical Psychology* 53:890-904.
Duhl, L.
  1986   The healthy city: its function and its future. *Health Promotion* 1:55-60.
Dwore, R.B., and M.W. Kreuter
  1980   Reinforcing the case for health promotion. *Family and Community Health* 2:103-119.
Dwyer, T., J.P. Pierce, C.D. Hannam, and N. Burke
  1986   Evaluation of the Sydney "Quit. For Life" anti-smoking campaign: part II: changes in smoking prevalence. *Medical Journal of Australia* 144:344-347.
Easterby-Smith, M.
  1986   *Evaluation of Management Education, Training and Development.* Brookfield, Vt.: Gower Publishing Co.
Farquhar, J.W.
  1978   The community-based model of life style intervention trials. *American Journal of Epidemiology* 108:103-111.

Farquhar, J.W., S.P. Fortmann, P.D. Wood, and W.L. Haskell
1983   Community studies of cardiovascular disease prevention. Pp. 170-182 in N.M. Kaplan and J. Stamler, eds., *Prevention of Coronary Heart Disease: Practical Management of Risk Factors*. Philadelphia, Pa.: W.B. Saunders Co.

Farquhar, J.W., S.P. Fortmann, J.A. Flora, C.B. Taylor, W.L. Haskell, P.T. Williams, N. Maccoby, and P.D. Wood
1990   Effects of community-wide education on cardiovascular disease risk factors—the Stanford 5-city Project. *Journal of the American Medical Association* 264:359-365.

Feighery, E., and T. Rogers
1990   Building and maintaining effective coalitions. *How-To Guides on Community Health Promotion*. Palo Alto, Calif.: Health Promotion Resource Center, Stanford Center for Research on Disease Prevention.

Fielding, J.E.
1982   Preventive medicine and the bottom line. *Journal of Occupational Medicine* 24:907-916.

Fielding, J.E., and L. Breslow
1983   Health promotion programs sponsored by California employers. *American Journal of Public Health* 73:538-542.

Fiore, M.C., T.E. Novotny, J.P. Pierce, E.J. Hatziandreu, K.M. Patel, and R.M. Davis
1989   Trends in cigarette smoking in the United States: the changing influence of gender and race. *Journal of the American Medical Association* 261:49-55.

Fitz-enz, J.
1984   *How to Measure Human Resources Management*. New York: McGraw-Hill.

Flay, B.R.
1986   Mass media linkages with school-based programs for drug abuse prevention. *Journal of School Health* 56:402-406.

Flay, B.R.
1987a   Social psychological approaches to smoking prevention: review and recommendations. Pp. 121-180 in *Advances in Health Education and Promotion*, Vol. 2. Greenwich, Conn.: JAI Press Inc.

Flay, B.R.
1987b   *Selling the Smokeless Society: 56 Evaluated Mass Media Programs and Campaigns Worldwide*. Washington, D.C.: American Public Health Association.

Food Marketing Institute
1989   *Trends: Consumer Attitudes and the Supermarket*. Washington, D.C.: Food Marketing Institute.

Freudenberg, N.
1984   *Not in Our Backyards! Community Action for Health*. New York: Monthly Review Press.

Gaziano, C.
1985   Neighborhood newspapers and neighborhood leaders: influences on agenda setting and definitions of issues. *Communication Research* 12:568-594.

Glanz, K., F.M. Lewis, and B.K. Rimer, eds.
1990   *Health Behavior and Health Education: Theory, Research, and Practice*. San Francisco: Jossey-Bass.

Glynn, T.J.
1981   Psychological sense of community: measurement and application. *Human Relations* 34:789-818.

Glynn, T.J.
1989   Essential elements of school-based smoking prevention programs. *Journal of School Health* 59:181-188.

Green, L.W.
    1970a   Should health education abandon attitude-change strategies? Perspectives from recent research. *Health Education Monographs* 1(30):25-48.

Green, L.W.
    1970b   *Status Identity and Preventive Health Behavior.* Berkeley, Calif.: Pacific Health Education Reports No. 1, University of California School of Public Health.

Green, L.W.
    1977   Evaluation and measurement: some dilemmas for health education. *American Journal of Public Health* 67:155-161.

Green, L.W.
    1986   The theory of participation: a qualitative analysis of its expression in national and international health policies. Pp. 211-236 in W. Ward, ed., *Advances in Health Education and Health Promotion*, Vol. 1. Greenwich, Conn.: JAI Press.

Green, L.W.
    1990   The revival of community and the public obligation of academic health centers. Pp. 148-164 in R. Bulger, R.E. Bulger, and S. Reiser, eds., *The Role of the Academic Health Center in Humanizing Medicine.* Ames, Iowa: University of Iowa Press.

Green, L.W., and A.L. McAlister
    1984   Macro-intervention to support health behavior: some theoretical perspectives and practical reflections. *Health Education Quarterly* 11(3):323-339.

Green, L.W., and M.W. Kreuter
    1991   *Health Promotion Planning: An Educational and Environmental Approach.* Palo Alto, Calif.: Mayfield.

Green, L.W., and J. Raeburn
    1988   Health promotion: what is it? What will it become? *Health Promotion International* 3:151-159.

Green, L.W., P. Heit, D.C. Iverson, L.J. Kolbe, and M. Kreuter
    1980   The School Health Curriculum Project: its theory, practice and measurement experience. *Health Education Quarterly* 7:14-34.

Green, L.W., P.D. Mullen, and S. Maloney, eds.
    1984   Large-scale health education campaigns. *Health Education Quarterly* 11: whole issue 3.

Green, L.W., N.H. Gottlieb, and G. Parcel
    1991   Diffusion theory extended and applied. In W. Ward and F.M. Lewis, eds., *Advances in Health Education and Promotion*, Vol. 3. London: Jessica Kingsley Publishers.

Greene, J.C., R. Louis, and S.J. Wycoff
    1990   Preventive dentistry. II. Peridontal diseases, malocclusion, trauma, and oral cancer. *Journal of the American Medical Association* 263:421-425.

Gunn, W.J., D.C. Iverson, and M. Katz
    1985   Design of the school health education evaluation. *Journal of School Health* 55:301-304.

Haynes, R.B., D.W. Taylor, and D.L. Sackett, eds.
    1979   *Compliance in Health Care.* Baltimore, Md.: Johns Hopkins University Press.

Hertel, V.
    1982   Changing times in school nursing. *Journal of School Health* 52:313-314.

Holder, H.D.
    1991   *Community Prevention Trials for Alcohol Problems: Methodological Issues.* New York: Praeger.

Holder, H., and N. Giesbrecht
  1989   Conceptual issues: perspectives on the community in action research. Pp. 27-40
          in N. Giesbrecht, P. Conley, R. W. Denniston, L. Gliksman, H. Holder, A. Pederson,
          R. Room, and M. Shain, eds. *Research, Action, and the Community: Experiences
          in the Prevention of Alcohol and Other Drug Problems.* Office of Substance
          Abuse Prevention Monograph 4, DHHS Pub. No. (ADM) 89-1651. Rockville,
          Md: Office for Substance Abuse Prevention.

Hunt, S.
  1990   Building alliances: professional and political issues in community participation:
          examples from a community development project. *Health Promotion Interven-
          tions* 5:179-185.

Israel, B.A.
  1985   Social networks and social support: implications for natural helper and commu-
          nity level interventions. *Health Education Quarterly* 12:65-80.

Jernigan, D.H., and J.F. Mosher
  1987   Preventing alcohol-related motor vehicle crashes: a policy agenda for the nation.
          Contemporary Drug Problems 14:243-278.

Katzman, M.S., and K.J. Smith
  1989   Evaluation of occupational health promotion programs. *Employee Assistance Quarterly*
          4(3):27-46.

King, J.A., L.L. Morris, and C.T. Fitz-Gibbon
  1987   *How to Assess Program Implementation.* Newbury Park, Calif.: Sage Publica-
          tions.

Kolbe, L.J.
  1982   What can we expect from school health education? *Journal of School Health*
          52:145-150.

Kolbe, L.J., and D.C. Iverson
  1980   Research in school health education: a needs assessment. Pp. 177-194 in *Pro-
          ceedings of the Planning Meeting on Cancer Education.* Bethesda, Md.: U.S.
          Department of Health, Education and Welfare.

Kolbe, L.J., and D.C. Iverson
  1983   Integrating school and community efforts to promote health: strategies, policies
          and methods. *Hygie: International Journal of Health Education* 3:40-47.

Kolbe, L.J., L.W. Green, J. Foreyt, L. Darnell, K. Goodrick, H. Williams, D. Ward, A.S.
        Korton, I. Karacan, R. Widmeyer, and G. Stainbrook
  1986   Appropriate functions of health education in schools: improving health and cogni-
          tive performance. Pp. 171-216 in N.A. Krasnegor, J.D. Arasteh, and M.F. Cataldo,
          eds., *Child Health Behavior: A Behavioral Pediatrics Perspective.* New York:
          Wiley.

Kotler, P., and E.L. Roberto
  1989   *Social Marketing: Strategies for Changing Public Behavior.* New York: The
          Free Press.

Kottke, T.E., P. Puska, J.T. Solomen, et al.
  1985   Projected effects of high-risk versus population-based prevention strategies in coronary
          heart disease. *American Journal of Epidemiology* 121:697-704.

Kreuter, M.W., and P.A. Reagan
  1980   Health education: coming of age in the schools. Pp. 75-95 in *Proceedings of the
          Planning Meeting on Cancer Education.* Bethesda, Md.: U.S. Department of
          Health and Human Services.

Kreuter, M.W., G.M. Christenson, and A. Divencenzo
  1982   The multiplier effect of the health education risk reduction grants program in 28
          states and 1 territory. *Public Health Reports* 97:510-515.

Lando, H.A., B. Loken, B. Howard-Pitney, and T. Pechacek
  1990a   Community impact of a localized smoking cessation contest. *American Journal of Public Health* 80:601-603.
Lando, H.A., P.G. McGovern, F.X. Barrios, and B.D. Etringer
  1990b   Comparative evaluation of American Cancer Society and American Lung Association smoking cessation clinics. *American Journal of Public Health* 80:554-559.
Lasater, T., D. Abrams, L. Artz, P. Beaudin, L. Cabrera, J. Elder, A. Ferreira, P. Knisley, G. Peterson, A. Rodriques, P. Rosenberg, R. Snow, and R. Carleton
  1984   Lay volunteer delivery of a community-based cardiovascular risk factor change program: the Pawtucket Experiment. Pp. 1166-1170 in J.D. Matarazzo, S.M. Weiss, J.A. Herd, N.E. Miller, and S.M. Weiss, eds., *Behavioral Health: A Handbook of Health Enhancement and Disease Prevention.* New York: John Wiley and Sons.
Lawrence, R.S.
  1990   The role of the physician in promoting health. *Health Affairs* 9:122-132.
Levit, K.R., and C.A. Cowan
‘ 1991   Business, households, and governments: health care costs, 1990. *Health Care Financing Report* 13:83-93.
Leviton, L.C., and R.O. Valdiser
  1990   Evaluating AIDS prevention: outcome, implementation, and mediating variables. *Evaluation and Program Planning* 13:55-66;
Light, L., and I.R. Contento
  1989   Changing the course: a school nutrition and cancer education curriculum developed by the American Cancer Society and the National Cancer Institute. *Journal of School Health* 59:205-209.
Maloney, S.K., and J.C. Hersey
  1984   Getting messages on the air: findings from the 1982 alcohol abuse prevention campaign. *Health Education Quarterly* 11:273-292.
Manoff, R.K.
  1985   *Social Marketing: New Imperative for Public Health.* New York: Praeger.
Markland, R.E., and M.L. Vincent
  1990   Improving resource allocation in a teenage sexual risk reduction program. *Socio-Economic Planning Science* 24:35-48.
Matarazzo, J.D., S.M. Weiss, J.A. Herd, N.E. Miller, and S.M. Weiss, eds.
  1984   *Behavioral Health: A Handbook of Health Enhancement and Disease Prevention.* New York: Wiley.
McCoy, H.V., S.E. Dodds, and C. Nolan
  1990   AIDS intervention design for program evaluation: the Miami community outreach project. *Journal of Drug Issues* 20:223-243.
McDonald, P., and R. Estep
  1985   Prime time drug depictions. *Contemporary Drug Problems* 14:419-438.
McGinnis, J.M., D. Shopland, and C. Brown
  1987   Tobacco and health: trends in smoking and smokeless tobacco consumption in the United States. *Annual Review of Public Health* 8:441-467.
McMillan, D.W., and D.M. Chavis
  1986   Sense of community: a definition and theory. *Journal of Community Psychology* 14:6-23.
Mechanic, D.M., ed.
  1983   *Handbook of Health, Health Care, and the Health Professions.* New York: The Free Press.
Metropolitan Life Foundation
  1988   *An Evaluation of Comprehensive Health Education in American Public Schools.*

Louis Harris and Associates, conducted for the Metropolitan Life Foundation, New York. Study no. 874024.

Millar, W.J., and B.E. Naegele
1987   Time to Quit program. *Canadian Journal of Public Health* 78:109-111.

Minkler, M.
1989   Health education, health promotion and the open society: an historical perspective. *Health Education Quarterly* 16:17-30.

Minkler, M.
1990   Improving health through community organization. Pp. 257-287 in K. Glanz, F.M. Lewis, and B.K. Rimer, eds., *Health Behavior and Health Education*. San Francisco: Jossey-Bass.

Mullen, P.D., and J.G. Zapka
1982   *Guidelines for Health Promotion and Education Services in HMOs*. Washington, D.C.: U.S. Government Printing Office.

Nader, P.R., J.G. Sallis, T.L. Patterson, I.S. Abramson, J.W. Rupp, K.L. Senn, C.J. Atkins, B.E. Roppe, J.A. Morris, J.P. Wallace, and W.A. Vega
1989   A family approach to cardiovascular risk reduction: results from the San Diego Family Health Project. *Health Education Quarterly* 16:229-244.

National Research Council
1989   *Improving Risk Communication*. Washington, D.C.: National Academy Press.

National Research Council
1993   *Under the Influence: Drugs and the American Worker*. Committee on Drug Use in the Workplace, Commission on Behavioral and Social Sciences and Education. Washington, D.C.: National Academy Press (in press).

National Restaurant Association
1989   *Foodservice Industry Forecast*. Washington, D.C.: Malcolm M. Knapp Research.

Newman, I.M.
1980   Smoking cessation from an educational perspective. Pp. 97-126 in *Proceedings of the Planning Meeting on Cancer Education*. Bethesda, Md.: U.S. Department of Health, Education and Welfare.

Nutbeam, D., and J. Catford
1987   The Welsh Heart Programme evaluation strategy: progress, plans and possibilities. *Health Promotion* 2:5-18.

Oberschall, A.
1973   *Social Conflict and Social Movements*. Englewood Cliffs, N.J.: Prentice-Hall.

Office of Disease Prevention and Health Promotion
1990   Public health communication. In U.S. Department of Health and Human Services, *Prevention '89/'90: Federal Programs and Progress*. Washington, D.C.: U.S. Government Printing Office.

Olsen, L.K., R. Hambleton, R. Simon, D.B. Connell, R.R. Turner, D. Orenstein
1985   Development and application of the student test used in the school health education evaluation. *Journal of School Health* 55:309-315.

Orlandi, M.A.
1986   The diffusion and adoption of worksite health promotion innovations: an analysis of barriers. *Preventive Medicine* 15:522-536.

Orlandi, M.A., C. Landers, R. Weston, and N. Haley
1990   Adoption and diffusion of health promotion innovations. Pp. 288-313 in K. Glanz, F.M. Lewis, and B.K. Rimer, eds., *Health Behavior and Health Education: Theory, Research and Practice*. San Francisco, Calif.: Jossey-Bass.

O'Rourke, T.W., and D.B. Stone
1980   School health education: cancer prevention and control. Pp. 143-175 in *Proceed-

ings of the Planning Meeting on Cancer Education. Bethesda, Md.: U.S. Department of Health, Education and Welfare.

Ostrow, D.G.
1985   AIDS prevention through effective education. *Daedalus: Journal of the American Academy of Arts and Sciences* 118:229-254.

Ottoson, J.M., and L.W. Green
1987   Reconciling concept and context: a theory of implementation. *Advances in Health Education and Promotion* 2:339-368.

Owen, S.L., M.A. Kirkpatrick, S.W. Lavery, H.L. Gonser, S.R. Nelson, R.L. Davis, E.F. Mason, and D.B. Connell
1985   Selecting and recruiting health programs for the school health education evaluation. *Journal of School Health* 55:305-308.

Paehlke, R.C.
1989   *Environmentalism and the Future of Progressive Politics.* New Haven, Conn.: Yale University Press.

Parcel, G.S., and T. Baranowski
1981   Social learning theory and health education. *Health Education* 12(3):14-18.

Parcel, G.S., M.P. Eriksen, C.Y. Lovato, N.H. Gottlieb, S.G. Brink, and L.W. Green
1989a   The diffusion of school-based tobacco-use prevention programs: project description and baseline data. *Health Education Research* 4(1):111-124.

Parcel, G.S., W.C. Taylor, S.G. Brink, N. Gottlieb, K. Engquist, N.M. O'Hara, and M.P. Eriksen
1989b   Translating theory into practice: intervention strategies for the diffusion of a health promotion innovation. *Family and Community Health* 12(3):1-13.

Parkinson, R.S., and Associates, eds.
1982   *Managing Health Promotion in the Workplace: Guidelines for Implementation and Evaluation.* Palo Alto, Calif.: Mayfield.

Patton, C.
1985   *Sex and Germs: The Politics of AIDS.* Boston, Mass.: South End Press.

Pentz, M.A.
1986   Community organization and school liaisons: how to get programs started. *Journal of School Health* 56:382-388.

Pentz, M.A., C. Cormack, B. Flay, W.B. Hansen, C.A. Johnson
1986   Balancing program and research integrity in community drug abuse prevention: Project STAR approach. *Journal of School Health* 56:389-393.

Pentz, M.A., J.H. Dwyer, D.P. MacKinnon, B.R. Flay, W.B. Hansen, E.Y.I. Wang, and C.A. Johnson
1989   A multicommunity trial for primary prevention of adolescent drug abuse: effects on drug use prevalence. *Journal of the American Medical Association* 261:3259-3266.

Perry, C.L., ed.
1986   Special issue on community programs for drug abuse prevention. *Journal of School Health* 56(9):357-418.

Perry, C.L., R.V. Luepker, D.M. Murray, C. Kurth, R. Mullis, S. Crockett, and D.R. Jacobs, Jr.
1988   Parent involvement with children's health promotion: the Minnesota Home Team. *American Journal of Public Health* 78:1156-1160.

Pertschuk, M., and A. Erikson
1987   *Smoke Fighting: A Smoking Control Movement Building Guide.* New York: American Cancer Society.

Pertschuk, M., and W. Schaetzel
1989   *The People Rising: The Campaign Against the Bork Nomination.* New York: Thunder's Mouth Press.

Phillips, J.J.
1983   *Handbook of Training Evaluation and Measurement Methods.* Houston, Texas: Gulf Publishing Co.

Pierce, J.P., M.C. Fiore, T.E. Novotny, E.J. Hatziandreu, and R.M. Davis
1989   Trends in cigarette smoking in the United States: educational differences are increasing. *Journal of the American Medical Association* 261:56-60.

Pierce, J.P., P. Macaskill, and D. Hill
1990   Long-term effectiveness of mass media led antismoking campaigns in Australia. *American Journal of Public Health* 80:565-569.

Pollock, M., and K. Middleton
1989   *Elementary School Health Instruction,* 2nd ed. St. Louis, Mo.: Times Mirror/ Mosby College Publishing.

Popkin, B., P. Haines, K. Reidy
1989   Food consumption trends of U.S. women: patterns and determinants between 1977 and 1985. *American Journal of Clinical Nutrition* 49:1307-1319.

Portnoy, B., D.M. Anderson, and M.P. Eriksen
1989   Application of diffusion theory to health promotion research. *Family and Community Health* 12(3):73-81.

Protess, D.L., D.R. Leff, S. Brooks, and M.T. Gordon
1985   Uncovering rape: the watchdog press and the limits of agenda setting. *Public Opinion Quarterly* 49:19-37.

Puska, P., A. McAlister, J. Pekkola, and K. Koskela
1981   Television in health promotion: evaluation of a national programme in Finland. *International Journal of Health Education* 24:2-14.

Puska, P., A. Nissinen, J. Tuomilehto, J.T. Salonen, K. Koskela, A. McAlister, T.E. Kottke, N. Maccoby, and J.W. Farquhar
1985   The community-based strategy to prevent coronary heart disease: conclusions from the ten years of the North Karelia Project. *Annual Review of Public Health* 6:147-193.

Reid, W.J., and P. Hanrahan
1988   Measuring implementation of social treatment. In K.J. Conrad and C. Roberts-Gray, eds., *Evaluating Program Environments.* San Francisco, Calif.: Jossey-Bass.

Resnick, L.B.
1987   *Education and Learning to Think.* Washington, D.C.: National Academy Press.

Riger, S., and P.J. Lavraka
1981   Community ties: patterns of attachment and social interaction in urban neighborhoods. *American Journal of Community Psychology* 9:55-66.

Rimer, B.K.
1990   Perspectives on intrapersonal theories in health education and health behavior. Pp. 140-157 in K. Glanz, F.M. Lewis, and B.K. Rimer, eds., *Health Behavior and Health Education: Theory, Research, and Practice.* San Francisco, Calif.: Jossey-Bass.

Room, R.
1989   Introduction—community action and alcohol problems: the demonstration project as an unstable mixture. Pp. 1-25 in Giesbrecht, P. Conley, R.W. Denniston, et al., eds., *Research, Action, and the Community: Experiences in the Prevention of Alcohol and Other Drug Problems.* Office of Substance Abuse Prevention Monograph 4, DHHS Publ. No (ADM) 89-1651. Rockville, Md.: Office for Substance Abuse Prevention.

Rothman, J., and E.R. Brown
  1989   Indicators of societal action to promote social health. Pp. 202-220 in S.B. Kar, ed., *Health Promotion Indicators and Actions*. New York: Springer Publishing Co.
Samuels, S.E.
  1990   Project LEAN: a national campaign to reduce dietary fat consumption. *American Journal of Health Promotion* 4:435-40.
Scheirer, M.A.
  1990   The life cycle of an innovation: adoption versus discontinuation of the fluoride mouth rinse program in schools. *Journal of Health and Social Behavior* 31:203-215.
Schiller, P., A. Steckler, L. Dawson, and F. Patton
  1987   *Participatory Planning in Community Health Education: A Guide Based on the McDowell County, West Virginia, Experience*. Oakland, Calif.: Third Party Associates.
Schorr, L.B.
  1989   *Within Our Reach: Breaking the Cycle of Disadvantage*. New York: Anchor Books, Doubleday.
Shaw, D.L., and M.E. McCombs
  1989   Dealing with illicit drugs: the power—and limits—of mass media agenda setting. Pp. 113-120 in P.J. Shoemaker, ed., *Communication Campaigns About Drugs: Government, Media, and the Public*. Hillsdale, N.J.: Lawrence Erlbaum Associates.
Shoemaker, P.J., ed.
  1989   *Communication Campaigns About Drugs: Government, Media, and the Public*. Hillsdale, N.J.: Lawrence Erlbaum Associates.
Simons-Morton, D.G., B.G. Simons-Morton, G.S. Parcel, and J.G. Bunker
  1988   Influencing personal and environmental conditions for community health: a multi-level intervention model. *Family and Community Health* 11:25-35.
Solomon, M.Z., and W. DeJong
  1986   Recent sexually transmitted disease prevention efforts and their implications for AIDS health education. *Health Education Quarterly* 13:301-316.
Spretnak, C., and F. Capra
  1984   *Green Politics*. New York: E.P. Dutton, Inc.
Staropoli, C.J., and C.F. Waltz
  1978   *Developing and Evaluating Educational Programs for Health Care Providers*. Philadelphia: F.A. Davis Co.
Stone, E.J., C.L. Perry, and R.V. Luepker
  1989   Synthesis of cardiovascular behavioral research for youth health promotion. *Health Education Quarterly* 16(2):155-169.
Terre, L., R.S. Drabman, and E.F. Meydrech
  1990   Relationships among children's health-related behaviors: a multivariate, developmental perspective. *Preventive Medicine* 19:134-146.
Thompson, B., and S. Kinne
  1990   Social change theory: applications to community health. Pp. 45-65 in N. Bracht, ed., *Health Promotion at the Community Level*. Newbury Park, Calif.: Sage.
U.S. Preventive Services Task Force
  1989   *Guide to Clinical Preventive Services: An Assessment of the Effectiveness of 169 Interventions*. Baltimore, Md.: Williams & Wilkins.
Vartiainen, E., P. Puska, L. Tossavainen, L. Viri, E. Niskanen, S. Moisio, A. McAlister, and U. Pallonen
  1986   Prevention of non-communicable diseases: risk factors in youth, the North Karelia Youth Project (1984-1988). *Health Promotion* 1:269-283.

Wallack, L.
1984   Drinking and driving: toward a broader understanding of the role of mass media. *Journal of Public Health Policy* 5:471-496.
Wallack, L.
1990   Media advocacy: promoting health through mass communication. Chap. 16 in K. Glanz, F.M. Lewis, and B.K. Rimer, eds., *Health Behavior and Health Education: Theory, Research, and Practice*. San Francisco, Calif.: Jossey-Bass.
Wallack, L., and C.K. Atkin, eds.
1990   *Mass Media and Health*. Newbury Park, Calif.: Sage Publications.
Wallack, L., W. Breed, and J. Cruz
1987   Alcohol on prime-time television. *Journal of Studies on Alcohol* 48:33-38.
Warner, K.E., and H.A. Murt
1983   Premature deaths avoided by the antismoking campaign. *American Journal of Public Health* 73:672-677.
Williams, L.S.
1986   AIDS risk reduction: a community health education intervention for minority high risk group members. *Health Education Quarterly* 13:407-422.
Williams, R.M.
1990   Rx: social reconnaissance. *Foundation News* 31(4):24-29.
Winett, R.A., D.G. Altman, and A.C. King
1990   Conceptual and strategic foundations for effective media campaigns for preventing the spread of HIV infection. *Evaluation and Program Planning* 13:91-104.
Young, J.
1981   The amplification of drug use. In S. Cohen and J. Young, eds., *The Manufacture of News*. London: Constable.

Index